51 Plant-Based High-Protein Recipes

For Athletic Performance and Muscle Growth

By Jules Neumann
Version 1.1
Published by HMPL Publishing
Get to know your publisher and related work at
happyhealthygreen.life

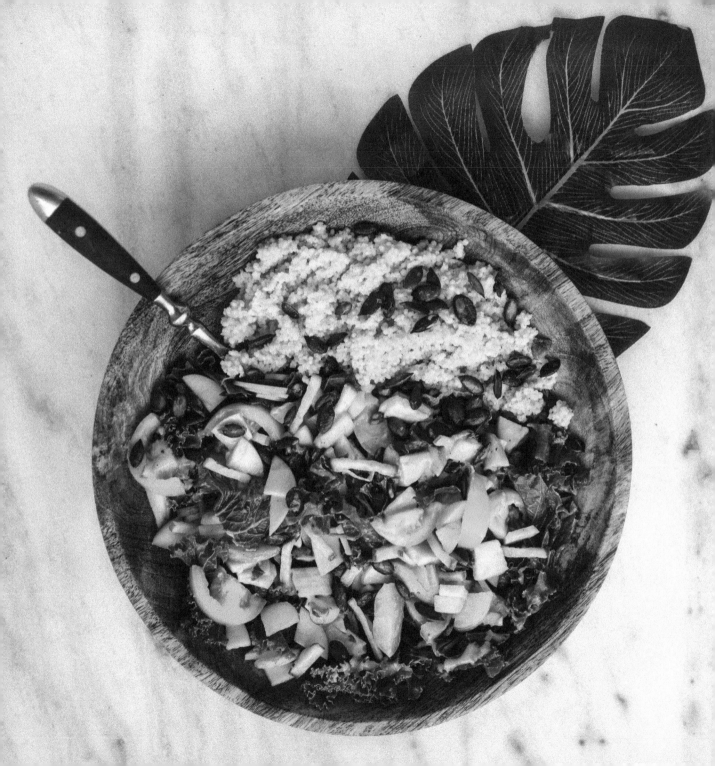

Introduction

These 51 plant-based, high-protein recipes will help you create a diet regimen that guarantees that your body gets enough protein each day. The dishes in this book will also make it easier for you to achieve your fitness goals. By eating a well-rounded diet with enough protein, you're one step closer to building the body of your dreams.

Protein is important for more than just recovery and muscle growth. The essential macronutrient is also required for the production and availability of hormones in the body. Following a diet with a balanced amino acid profile is critical for everyone, but even more so if you're physically active or following an intense exercise regimen.

All recipes in this book include serving sizes, storage information, and obviously, calorie, protein, carb, and fat content. Make sure to buy all ingredients before you start cooking. Then get ready to enjoy these 51 tasty dishes high in protein!

Table of Contents

Disclaimer

The recipes provided in this report are for informational purposes only and are not intended to provide dietary advice. A medical practitioner should be consulted before making any changes in your diet. Additionally, recipe cooking times may require adjustment depending on age and quality of appliances. Readers are strongly urged to take all precautions to ensure ingredients are fully cooked in order to avoid the dangers of foodborne viruses. The recipes and suggestions provided in this book are solely the opinion of the author. The author and publisher do not take any responsibility for any consequences that may result due to following the instructions provided in this book.

Congratulations on your responsible and health-conscious decision to read this book.

We're grateful you've joined us and excited for your journey ahead.

We offer our readers the exclusive opportunity to become part of our readers' circle. Dozens of people are already enjoying *bonus* plant-based recipes and extra support on their journey to better cooking, meal-prepping, and weight loss (or gain, when intended).

Become part of our readers' circle today and get *The Vegan Cookbook* free of charge!

Simply subscribe to our newsletter and join hundreds of people with similar ethics and goals.

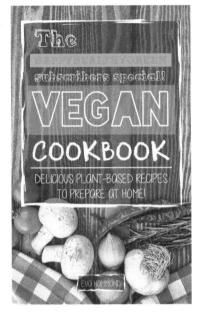

http://happyhealthygreen.life/about-us/evahammond/vegan-newsletter

By becoming part of our readers' circle, you will receive our latest recipes, useful articles, and many more tips to stay healthy, right in your inbox.

Our readers enjoy unique support in their health plans and can always reach out to us for personal questions.

http://happyhealthygreen.life/about-us/evahammond/vegan-newsletter

Subscribe and become part of our readers' circle and get instant access to our unique *The Vegan Cookbook*'!

Enter your email address and let us help you stay committed.

Choose the plant-based lifestyle and renounce animal cruelty. **See you inside the readers' circle!**

**We hate spam and will never email you more than twice a week.

Soaking methods & cooking recipes for plant-based staple foods

These ingredients are ideal for adding texture, flavor, fiber, protein, or just a base to your meals.

SOAKING

Beans, lentils, and split peas are rich in protein and fiber, but anti-nutrients found in beans and lentils prevent nutrient absorption in the gut. Soaking these ingredients in water and then rinsing them is an efficient way to eliminate anti-nutrients and ensure your body can take advantage of the full nutrient content of your diet. Another method to achieve this is sprouting. Both are explained in the tables below.

OVERNIGHT SOAK

Leaving beans, lentils, and legumes in a pot of water overnight (for at least 8 hours) is the most effective way to soak them. Use roughly 10 cups of water for every pound of dry beans (roughly 2 cups). Required soaking times are shown in the table below.

HOT SOAK

This is the quickest soaking method. Fill up a pot large enough to accommodate your beans or legumes with water. Add about 10 cups for each pound (roughly 2 cups) of dry beans, or simply ensure beans/legumes are covered with an excess of about 1 inch of water. Bring the water to a boil and allow it to simmer for about 3 minutes. Remove the pot from the heat, cover, and allow it to sit for 1 to 4 hours.

RINSING

After soaking, use a colander to drain the water from the pot and rinse the beans or legumes once or twice with fresh, cool water. This will wash off most of the indigestible sugars and anti-nutrients.

Boiling

After soaking and rinsing, fill a large pot to accommodate your beans or legumes with an excess of 1 inch of water. Set your burner (or stove) to a low heat until the water reaches a medium boil. Partially cover the pot with a lid. Cook times vary according to the kind of bean or legume and are listed below.

Cannallini, white kidney, and red beans need boiling to get rid of poison.

Optionally, add acidic ingredients like lemon juice, vinegar, or wine after cooking and draining the beans to prevent them from becoming tender.

Soaking and cooking time per bean or legume

(Per 1 cup)	Soak Time (in hours)	Cook Time	Yield (in cups)
Azuki Beans	4	45-55 min.	3
Anasazi Beans	4-8	60 min.	2-1/4
Black Beans	4	60-90 min.	2-1/4
Black-Eyed Peas	-	60 min.	2
Cannellini Beans	8-12	60 min.	2
Fava Beans	8-12	40-50 min.	1-2/3
Chickpeas	6-8	1-3 hrs.	2
Great Northern Beans	8-12	1-1 ½ hrs.	2-2/3
Green Split Peas	-	45 min.	2
Yellow Split Peas	-	1-1 ½ hrs.	2
Green Peas (whole)	8-12	1-2 hrs.	2

(Per 1 cup)	Soak Time (in hours)	Cook Time	Yield (in cups)
Kidney Beans	6-8	60 min.	2-1/4
Lentils, brown	8-12	45-60 min.	2-1/4
Lentils, green	8-12	30-45 min.	2
Lentils (red or yellow)	8-12	20-30 min.	2 to 2-1/2
Lima Beans (large)	8-12	45-60 min.	2
Lima Beans (small)	8-12	50-60 min.	3
Mung Beans	-	60 min.	2
Navy Beans	6-8	45-60 min.	2-2/3
Pink Beans	4-8	50-60 min.	2-3/4
Pinto Beans	6-8	1-1 ½ hrs.	2-2/3
Soybeans	8-12	1-2 hrs.	3
Tepary Beans	8-12	90 min.	3

*The recommended times in this chart are approximate.

A pressure cooker will reduce the amount of cook time needed. A 15-pound pressure cooker will reduce cooking time by 600%. In other words, what would normally take 1 hour, takes only 10 minutes with a pressure cooker. Adding Kombu seaweed to an overnight soak also speeds up cooking time by about 200%.

To test whether your beans are ready to be eaten, remove one from the pot, allow it to cool and place it between your tongue and the roof of your mouth. Apply pressure with your tongue. If it "smooshes" easily, the beans are ready.

SPROUTING

An alternative to soaking is sprouting. This means activating germination in a seed. It takes longer than soaking, but makes the nutrients in the seed more available for absorption. The process effectively reduces the anti-nutrient phytate by 37-81%, depending on the type of grain or legume.

Start by rinsing the seeds and placing them in cold water for 2-12 hours. After soaking, rinse the seeds again. Then place the soaked seeds into a sprouter for the appropriate length of time for that bean or seed. If you don't have a sprouter, a deep plate covered by a lid or towel works. Rinse the seeds every 8 to 12 hours. When the beans, grains, or legumes have sprouted a root, they are ready to be cooked.

Below is a list of sprouting times for various nuts, beans, legumes, seeds, and grains:

- Almond: 12 hours
- Adzuki beans: 3-5 days
- Chickpea: 12 hours
- Lentil: 12 hours
- Kamut: 2-3 days
- Wheat: 2-3 days
- Oats: 2-3 days
- Spelt & Rye: 2-3 days
- Barley: 2 days
- Buckwheat: 1-2 days
- Quinoa: 1-2 days

- Millet: 2-3 days
- Rice: 3-5 days
- Corn: 2-3 days
- Pepita: 1-2 days
- Fenugreek: 3-5 days
- Black beans: 3 days
- White beans: 2-3 days
- Mung beans: 2-5 days
- Kidney beans: 5-7 days
- Navy beans: 2-3 days
- Peas: 2-3 days

- Amaranth grains: 1-3 days
- Wheat berries: 3-4 days
- Wild rice: 3-5 days
- Black rice: 3-5 days
- Radish seeds: 3-4 days
- Alfalfa seeds: 3-5 days
- Pumpkin seeds: 1-2 days
- Sesame seeds: 1-2 days
- Sunflower seeds: 2-3 days

Soaking and sprouting chia, hemp and flaxseeds

Like with other seeds, soaking chia, hemp, and flaxseeds help to maximize nutrient availability and seed digestibility, but the process is a little different for these smaller seeds, which have a mucilaginous coating. When left in water, the coating starts to dissolve and creates a gel-like mixture.

To soak chia seeds, place seeds in a jar or sealed container and add water. Shake it for 2-3 minutes and place the container in the fridge. To fully soak the seeds, refrigerate for at least 1 hour, but an overnight soak is ideal in order to achieve the gel-like consistency of the mixture you are aiming for.

Tip: Use a mason jar so that seeds can be kept in the fridge for longer periods. Since this seed does not go bad easily, it is possible to always have some ready in the fridge.

Hemp seeds are one of the most easily digested plant protein sources, and do not require soaking—they can be consumed dry.

Flaxseeds, on the other hand, are prepared in a similar way to chia seeds. Place them in a jar with water and shake before leaving them to soak for 10 minutes to 2 hours at room temperature. The water will turn opaque from the soluble fiber and gums being excreted from the seeds. This water can be re-used to cook with and will contribute additional nutrients to a meal.

Sprouting

Similarly, the process used to sprout smaller seeds like chia and flaxseed differs from that of larger seeds. Soak the seeds in a shallow dish and drain. Cover the dish with foil or move the seeds to a plastic bowl. Place the dish or bowl in a sunlit area and spray the seeds with water twice a day. After 3 to 7 days, the seeds will sprout.

Rice

Rice is a popular staple food and comes in many varieties. Each variety requires its own preparation method. Brown rice, for example, requires more water and takes longer to cook than white rice. You can prepare a range of healthy rice dishes using a rice cooker, pot, or steamer.

TYPES OF RICE:

- Long-grain rice – fluffy grains that stay separated (basmati, jasmine, red cargo)
- Medium-grain rice – tender, moist, and chewy (brown, rosematta)
- Short-grain rice – short and plump, stick together and clump up (sticky, sushi, Valencia)

It is a good idea to rinse rice (except short-grain rice) prior to cooking to remove excess starch. For short-grain rice, the starch provides the desired texture for the dishes in which it's commonly used.

COOKING IN A POT

METHOD FOR LONG-GRAIN RICE:
1. Measure the rice into a cup and level the top.
2. Rinse the rice with cold water until the water is clear.
3. Optional: soak the rice for up to 30 minutes and drain. Doing so will remove surface starch and make the rice less sticky.
4. Pour the rinsed rice into a pot.
5. Add 2 cups of water for every 1 cup of dry rice.
6. Optional: add a pinch of salt and oil of choice.
7. Bring the water to a soft boil.
8. Put the lid on top of the pot and softly shake the pot to distribute the rice evenly.
9. Cook for 10 minutes with the lid on.
10. Once all water is absorbed, turn off the heat, remove the lid, and cover the pot with a tea towel.
11. Set aside to use in another recipe or serve and enjoy as is!

METHOD FOR MEDIUM-GRAIN RICE:
1. Measure the rice into a cup and level the top.
2. Rinse the rice in a strainer with cold water to improve texture and get rid of grit and dust that may be left in the uncooked rice.
3. Add 2 cups water for each cup of (brown) rice
4. Optional: add a little olive oil.
5. Bring the water to a boil, lower the heat, and cook the rice for 45 minutes.
6. Check the rice. The majority of water should be gone – a little left is fine.
7. Drain excess water if necessary.
8. After cooking, allow the rice to sit with the lid on for about 10 minutes.

9. Fluff the rice with a fork and transfer it to a dish.
10. Set aside for use in another recipe or consume and enjoy as is!

METHOD FOR SHORT-GRAIN RICE:

1. Measure the rice into a cup and level the top.
2. Wash the rice with a small amount of cold water to get rid of grit and dust that may be left in the uncooked rice.
3. Fill a pot with equal parts water and rice.
4. Soak the rice for at least 15 minutes or up to 3 hours.
5. Cover the pot and bring the water to a boil.
6. Once the water is boiling, turn the heat to low.
7. Allow the rice to simmer for about 15 minutes without removing the lid.
8. When all the water is absorbed, you'll hear a hissing sound.
9. Turn off the heat, allow the rice to stand covered with the lid for 10 to 20 minutes.
10. Remove the lid and set the rice aside for another recipe or serve and enjoy!

Recommended rice-water ratios for different grain types.

Type of rice	Water needed
White, long grain	1 ¾ - 2 cups per 1 cup rice
White, medium grain	1 ½ cups per 1 cup rice
White, short grain	1 ¼ cups per 1 cup rice
Brown, long grain	2 ¼ cups per 1 cup rice
Brown, medium grain	2 cups per 1 cup rice

For rice that is usually served dry (e.g. Basmati or Jasmin), use slightly less water than designated above.

COOKING IN A RICE COOKER

A rice cooker is device bit like a slow cooker that adjusts cook time to different types of rice and keeps it warm after it is ready. Preparation steps for using a rice cooker are otherwise the same as described for cooking with a standard pot.

QUINOA

Quinoa is common in many vegan recipes since it is a complete protein, containing all the essential amino acids. It's great for curries or salads. This superfood is easy to cook and, like rice, comes in several different varieties such as white, red, and black. White quinoa carries the most neutral flavor, while red and black have more distinct flavors and are often used in salads.

METHOD FOR PREPARING QUINOA:

1. Measure the quinoa into a cup and level the top.
2. Thoroughly rinse the quinoa in a strainer with cold water and drain.
3. Add 2 cups water for each cup of quinoa
4. Bring the water to a boil.
5. Optional: occasionally stir the quinoa with a wooden spoon.
6. Cover the pot with a lid.
7. Turn the heat low and allow the quinoa to simmer for 15 minutes.
8. Remove the pot from the heat and let the quinoa sit with the lid on for 5 to 10 minutes.
9. Remove the lid, fluff, and set aside or serve and enjoy!

ESSENTIALS

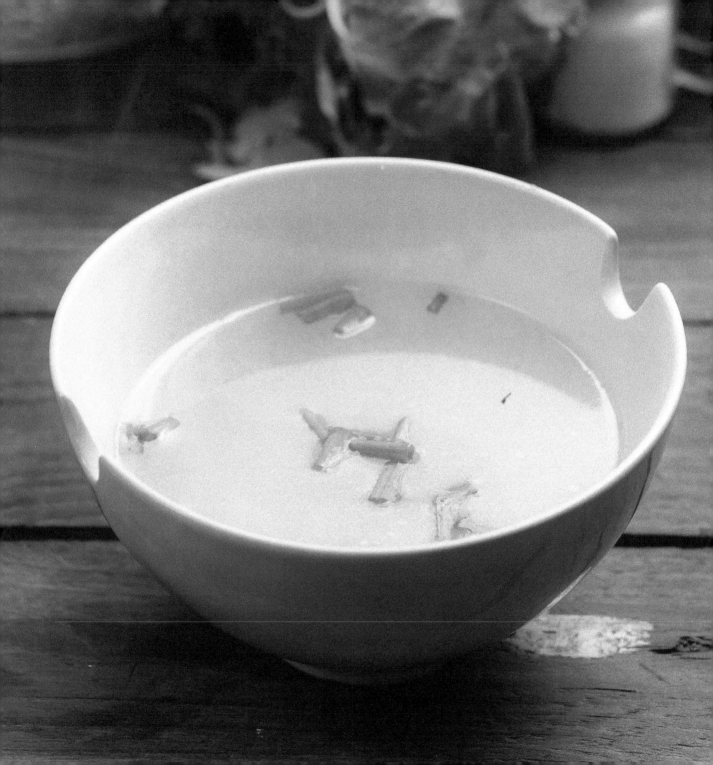

1. Vegetable Broth

Serves: 5 cups
| Prep Time: ~120 min |

Nutrition Information
(per serving)
- Calories: 0 kcal.
- Carbs: 0g.
- Fat: 0g.
- Protein: 0g.
- Fiber: 0g.
- Sugar: 0g.

INGREDIENTS:

- 10 cups water
- 2 onions (chopped)
- 3 cloves garlic (medium, minced)
- 4 carrots (chopped)
- 3 celery ribs (leafless, chopped)
- 1 sweet potato (cubed)
- 1 red bell pepper (sliced)
- 1 cup kale (fresh or frozen, cut)
- ½ cup parsley (fresh)
- ½ cup olive oil
- 1 tbsp. miso paste
- 2 tbsp. nutritional yeast (optional)
- 1 tbsp. thyme
- 1 tbsp. rosemary
- Salt and black pepper to taste

Total number of ingredients: 15

METHOD:

1. Preheat oven at 400°F or 200°C.
2. Toss the onions, garlic, carrots, celery, sweet potato, bell pepper, kale and parsley with the ½ cup of olive oil in an oven-proof roasting pan or baking tray.
3. Bake the veggies in the oven for about 20 minutes until browned and caramelized.
4. Put a large pot over medium heat and boil about 10 cups of water.
5. Add all ingredients from the roasting pan to the pot with boiling water.
6. Immediately bring the heat down to low and keep it at boiling point.
7. Stir every few minutes and add the miso paste, nutritional yeast, thyme and rosemary.
8. Add salt, pepper and any other desired spices to taste.
9. Cook until half of the water has evaporated.
10. Take the pot off the stove and let it cool.
11. Pour the mixture through a sieve and collect the broth in a second pot. Don't waste the veggies afterwards, it makes for a nice side dish.
12. Use or store!

STORAGE INFORMATION:

Storage	Temperature	Expiration date	Preparation
Airtight container L	Fridge at 38 – 40°F or 3°C	5 days after preparation	Reheat in microwave or pot
Airtight container L	Freezer at -1°F or -20°C	60 days after preparation	Thaw at room temperature. Reheat in microwave or pot

When freezing, divide the broth into smaller portions for convenient use.

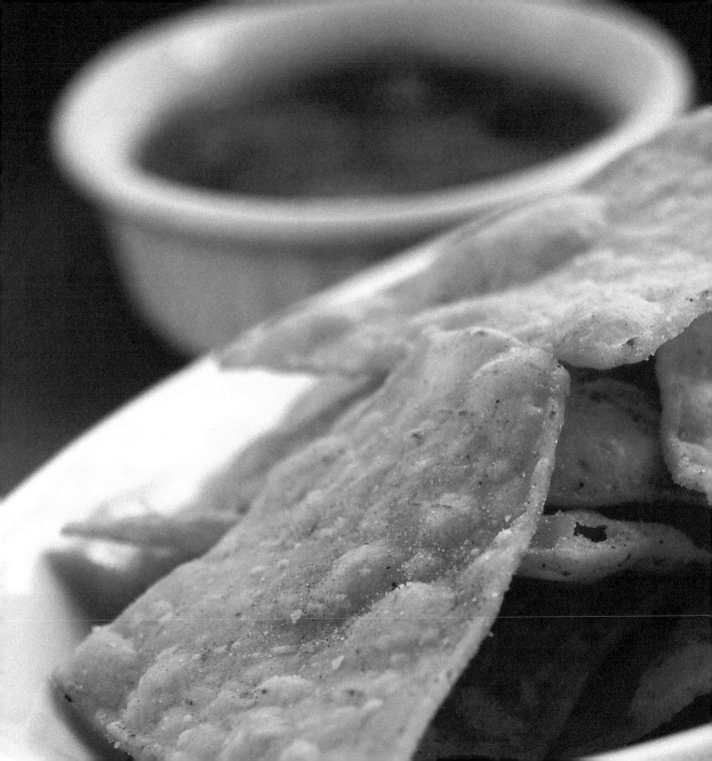

2. Mexican Salsa

Serves: 6 | Prep Time: ~5 min |

Nutrition Information
(per serving)

- Calories: 30 kcal.
- Carbs: 6.1g.
- Fat: 0.3g.
- Protein: 0.8g.
- Fiber: 2.1g.
- Sugar: 4.2g.

INGREDIENTS:

- 4 firm tomatoes (large)
- 1 fresh jalapeno·
- 2 tbsp. fresh cilantro (chopped)
- ½ red onion (medium, diced)
- 1 lime
- Salt and black pepper to taste

Total number of ingredients: 6

METHOD:

1. Skin and seed the tomatoes. Halve the jalapeno and remove the stem, seeds and placenta.
2. Cut the tomatoes and jalapeno into fine pieces.
3. Add the cut veggies to a medium size bowl.
4. Chop the cilantro and red onion into tiny bits and add to the bowl.
5. Juice the lime into the bowl and stir the ingredients well.
6. Season the mixture to taste with salt and black pepper.
7. After all the ingredients are combined, let it sit in the fridge for one hour before serving.
8. Enjoy, share or store for later!

STORAGE INFORMATION:

Storage	Temperature	Expiration date	Preparation
Airtight containerS	Fridge at 38 – 40°F or 3°C	3-4 days after preparation	
Airtight containerS	Freezer at -1°F or -20°C	60 days after preparation	Thaw at room temperature.

3. Easy Baba Ganoush

Serves: 2 | Prep Time: ~15 min |

Nutrition Information
(per serving)
- Calories: 246 kcal.
- Carbs: 21.5g.
- Fat: 15.4g.
- Protein: 5.3g.
- Fiber: 8.3g.
- Sugar: 10.3g.

INGREDIENTS:
- 1 eggplant (large, sliced)
- 1 tbsp. MCT oil
- 4 tbsp. lemon juice
- 2 tbsp. tahini
- 2 garlic cloves (medium, minced)
- Salt and pepper to taste
- 2 tsp. sesame seeds (optional)
- Small carrot (optional, cut)
- Handful fresh cilantro, parsley or basil (optional, chopped)

Total number of ingredients: 9

METHOD:
1. Preheat oven to 400°F or 200°C.
2. Put the sliced eggplant on a baking sheet.
3. Drizzle both sides of the eggplant with the MCT oil.
4. Put the baking sheet on a rack in the oven.
5. Allow the eggplant slices to broil for 2 minutes on each side.
6. Take the tray out of the oven and sprinkle the eggplant slices with salt.
7. Cover the tray with aluminum foil and put it back into the oven and allow the slices to steam for about 4 minutes.
8. Unwrap the eggplant, peel off its skin and transfer the eggplant to a blender.
9. Add the lemon juice, tahini, garlic, salt and pepper to taste and blend until smooth.
10. Transfer the mixture to a medium size bowl.
11. Top the baba ganoush with two or three of the optional ingredients.
12. Enjoy or store!

STORAGE INFORMATION:

Storage	Temperature	Expiration date	Preparation
Airtight container M/L	Fridge at 38 – 40°F or 3°C	3 days after preparation	
Airtight container M/L	Freezer at -1°F or -20°C	60 days after preparation	Thaw at room temperature.

Tip: serve the baba ganoush with some fresh pita bread or grilled sweet potatoes

4. Marinara Sauce

Serves: 13 | Prep Time: ~40 min |

Nutrition Information
(per serving)
- Calories: 65 kcal
- Carbs: 4.9 g.
- Fat: 4.3 g.
- Protein: 1.5 g.
- Fiber: 1.3 g.
- Sugar: 3 g.

INGREDIENTS:
- 4 28-oz. cans diced tomatoes
- 1 cup fresh basil (chopped)
- 4 tbsp. olive oil
- 4 tbsp. nutritional yeast
- 6 medium garlic cloves (minced)
- 2 tsp. dried oregano
- 1½ tbsp. maple syrup
- ½ tsp. cayenne pepper
- Salt to taste

Total number of ingredients: 9

METHOD:
1. Heat a large pot over medium heat.
2. Add the olive oil and minced garlic; sauté for about 1 minute.
3. Continue by adding the diced tomatoes, maple syrup, cayenne pepper, and oregano. Taste and add salt accordingly.
4. Bring the mixture to a simmer. Reduce the heat to low and cover the pot. Simmer the ingredients for about 25 minutes.
5. Add the basil and nutritional yeast. Stir well. Add more water if necessary.
6. Add more spices or salt to taste.
7. Incorporate the sauce in a dish, or store for future use.

STORAGE INFORMATION:

Storage	Temperature	Expiration date	Preparation
Airtight container M	Fridge at 38 – 40°F or 3°C	4-5 days after preparation	
Airtight container M	Freezer at -1°F or -20°C	60 days after preparation	Thaw at room temperature

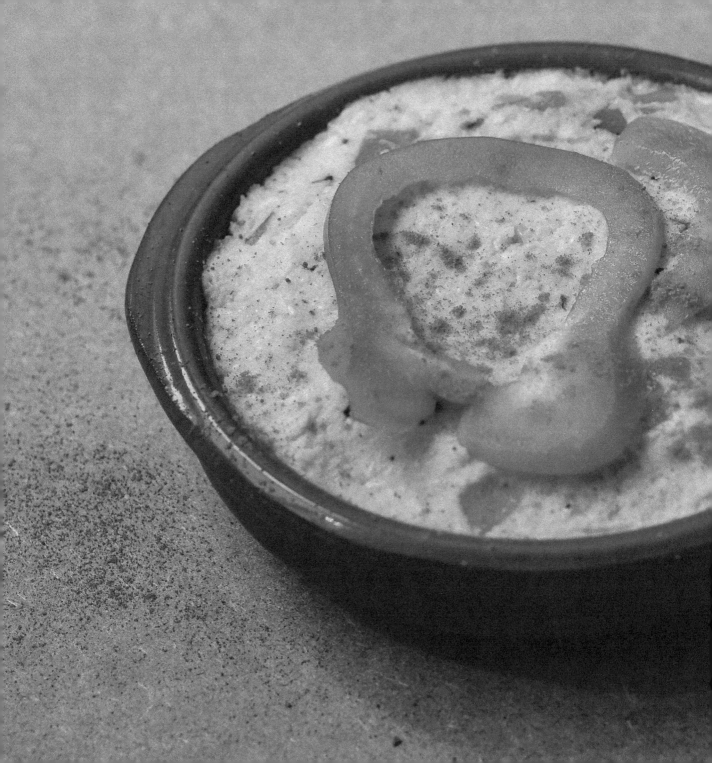

5. Hummus

Nutrition Information
(per serving)
- Calories: 97 kcal.
- Carbs: 13g.
- Fat: 3g.
- Protein: 4.6g.
- Fiber: 3.5g.
- Sugar: 2.5g.

INGREDIENTS:
- 3 cups of dry chickpeas
- 3 tbsp. olive oil
- 3 tbsp. tahini
- ½ cup water
- 3 tbsp. lemon juice (more to taste)
- ½ tsp. cumin
- Salt and pepper to taste

Total number of ingredients: 8

METHOD:
1. Preheat oven to 400°F or 200°C.
2. Prepare the chickpeas according to the "Soaking and cooking time per bean or legume" on page 7.
3. Add most of the cooked chickpeas, olive oil, tahini and the water to a blender.
4. Blend all the ingredients until all ingredients are incorporated and the hummus is smooth.
5. Transfer the hummus to a container and top it with some additional olive oil, cooked chickpeas and salt and pepper to taste.
6. Enjoy, share or store for later!

STORAGE INFORMATION:

Storage	Temperature	Expiration date	Preparation
Airtight container M/L	Fridge at 38 – 40°F or 3°C	4-5 days after preparation	
Airtight container M/L	Freezer at -1°F or -20°C	60 days after preparation	Thaw at room temperature.

6. Peanut Butter

Serves: 2 cups of peanut butter / 10 servings | Prep Time: ~15 minutes |

Nutrition Information (per serving)
 - Calories: 153 kcal.
 - Carbs: 7.8 g.
 - Fat: 11.4 g.
 - Protein: 4.8 g.
 - Fiber: 1.0 g.
 - Sugar: 1.7 g.

INGREDIENTS:
 - 2 cups raw peanuts (unsalted)
 - ½ tsp. sea salt

Total number of ingredients: 2

METHOD:
1. Preheat the oven to 375°F / 190°C.
2. Roast the peanuts for about 10 minutes.
3. Transfer them to a food processor and process for about 1 minute.
4. Scrape down the sides of the food processor, add the sea salt, and blend again for 1 minute; continue until the desired consistency is reached.
5. For the best flavor, chill the mix before serving.

STORAGE INFORMATION:

Storage	Temperature	Expiration date	Preparation
Airtight container S/M/L	Fridge at 38 – 40°F or 3°C	5 days after preparation	
Airtight container S/M/L	Freezer at -1°F or -20°C	60 days after preparation	Thaw at room temperature

7. Cashew Cheese Spread

Serves: 1 cup of cheese / 5 servings | Prep Time: ~5 min |

Nutrition Information
(per serving)

- Calories: 151kcal.
- Carbs: 8.8g.
- Fat: 10.9g.
- Protein: 4.6g.
- Fiber: 1.0g.
- Sugar: 1.7g.

INGREDIENTS:

- 1 cup water
- 1 cup raw cashews
- 1 tsp. nutritional yeast
- ½ tsp. salt
- 1 tsp. garlic powder (optional)

Total number of ingredients: 5

METHOD:

1. Soak the cashews for 6 hours in a medium-sized bowl filled with water.
2. Drain and transfer the soaked cashews to a food processor.
3. Add 1 cup water and all the other ingredients and blend.
4. For the best flavor, serve chilled.
5. Enjoy or store for later!

STORAGE INFORMATION:

Storage	Temperature	Expiration date	Preparation
Airtight container M	Fridge at 38 – 40°F or 3°C	4-5 days after preparation	
Airtight container M	Freezer at -1°F or -20°C	60 days after preparation	Thaw at room temperature.

8. Enchilada Sauce

Nutrition Information
(per serving)
- Calories: 18 kcal
- Carbs: 0.6 g.
- Fat: 1.6 g.
- Protein: 0.1 g.
- Fiber: 0.2 g.
- Sugar: 0.1 g.

INGREDIENTS:

- 1½ tbsp. MCT oil
- ½ tbsp. chili powder
- ½ tbsp. whole wheat flour
- ½ tsp. ground cumin
- ¼ tsp. oregano (dried or fresh)
- ¼ tsp. salt (or to taste)
- 1 garlic clove (minced)
- 1 tbsp. tomato paste
- 1 cup vegetable broth (page 17)
- ½ tsp. apple vinegar
- ½ tsp. ground black pepper

Total number of ingredients: 11

METHOD:

1. Heat a small saucepan over medium heat.
2. Add the MCT oil and minced garlic to the pan and sauté for about 1 minute.
3. Mix the dry spices and flour in a medium bowl and pour the dry mixture into the sauce pan.
4. Stir in the tomato paste immediately, and slowly pour in the vegetable broth, making sure that everything combines well.
5. When everything is mixed thoroughly, bring up the heat to medium-high until it gets to a simmer and cook for about 3 minutes or until the sauce becomes a bit thicker.
6. Remove the pan from the heat and add the vinegar with the black pepper, adding more salt and pepper to taste.

STORAGE INFORMATION:

Storage	Temperature	Expiration date	Preparation
Airtight container M	Fridge at 38 – 40°F or 3°C	4-5 days after preparation	
Airtight container M	Freezer at -1°F or -20°C	60 days after preparation	Thaw at room temperature

Tip: Add between 2 and 4 teaspoons of salt!

ENERGIZING BREAKFASTS

1. Cinnamon Apple Protein Smoothie

Nutrition Information
(per serving)
- Calories: 373 kcal
- Carbs: 21.7 g.
- Fat: 10.3 g.
- Protein: 48.5 g.
- Fiber: 3.5 g.
- Sugar: 12.2 g.

INGREDIENTS:
- 1 green apple (peeled, cored, and chopped)
- 1 cup coconut milk
- ½ tsp. cinnamon
- 2 scoops of vegan protein powder (vanilla flavor)
- 3 ice cubes (optional)
- 1-2 tsp. matcha powder (optional)

Total number of ingredients: 8

METHOD:
1. Add all the required, and optional (if desired), ingredients to a blender.
2. Blend for 2 minutes.
3. Transfer the shake to a large cup or shaker.
4. Top with some additional cinnamon powder or sticks.
5. Serve and enjoy!

STORAGE INFORMATION:

Storage	Temperature	Expiration date	Preparation
Ziploc bag	Fridge at 38 – 40°F or 3°C	2-3 days after preparation	
Ziploc bag	Freezer at -1°F or -20°C	30 days after preparation	

This is a classic taste in a vegan smoothie— perfect if you love the apple / cinnamon combination.

2. Tropical Protein Smoothie

Nutrition Information
(per serving)

- Calories: 350 kcal
- Carbs: 44.4 g.
- Fat: 6.7 g.
- Protein: 27.9 g.
- Fiber: 5.8 g.
- Sugar: 30.5 g.

INGREDIENTS:

- 1 orange (peeled and parted)
- 1 cup mango chunks (frozen or fresh)
- 1 banana (frozen or fresh)
- ½ cup blueberries
- 2 scoops of vegan protein powder (chocolate or vanilla flavor)
- 1 tbsp. hemp seeds
- 1 tsp. guarana (optional)
- 6 ice cubes

Total number of ingredients: 8

METHOD:

1. Add all the required ingredients, and the optional guarana (if desired), to a blender.
2. Blend for 2 minutes.
3. Transfer the shake to a large cup or shaker.
4. Enjoy!

STORAGE INFORMATION:

Storage	Temperature	Expiration date	Preparation
Ziploc bag	Fridge at 38 – 40°F or 3°C	2-3 days after preparation	
Ziploc bag	Freezer at -1°F or -20°C	30 days after preparation	

Tropical goodness in a smoothie, packed with carbs, minerals, vitamins, and protein— this one is also perfect as a pre-workout.

3. Cranberry Protein Shake

Serves: 3 | Prep Time: ~5 min |

Nutrition Information
(per serving)
- Calories: 325 kcal
- Carbs: 19.9 g.
- Fat: 16.8 g.
- Protein: 23.6 g.
- Fiber: 6.8 g.
- Sugar: 7.1 g.

INGREDIENTS:
- ¼ cup cranberries
- 2 scoops of vegan protein powder
  (chocolate or vanilla flavor)
- 1 banana (fresh or frozen)
- ¼ cup chia seeds
- ¼ cup hemp seeds
- 2 cups coconut milk
- 4 ice cubes

Total number of ingredients: 7

METHOD:
1. Soak the chia seeds according to the "Soaking and sprouting chia, hemp and flaxseeds" on page 10.
2. Add all ingredients to a blender.
3. Blend for 2 minutes.
4. Transfer to a large cup or shaker, and enjoy!

STORAGE INFORMATION:

Storage	Temperature	Expiration date	Preparation
Ziploc bag	Fridge at 38 – 40°F or 3°C	2-3 days after preparation	
Ziploc bag	Freezer at -1°F or -20°C	30 days after preparation	

Cranberry protein perfection... with healthy omega 3 fats and carbs to get that protein synthesis started, this smoothie is perfect as a post- workout.

4. Strawberry Orange Smoothie

Nutrition Information
(per serving)
- Calories: 287 kcal
- Carbs: 29.3 g.
- Fat: 7.5 g.
- Protein: 25.6 g.
- Fiber: 4.3 g.
- Sugar: 17.7 g.

INGREDIENTS:

- 2 cups coconut milk
- 10 strawberries (fresh or frozen)
- 1 orange (peeled and parted)
- 1 banana (fresh or frozen)
- 3 scoops of vegan protein powder
  (vanilla flavor)
- 2 ice cubes (optional)

Total number of ingredients: 6

METHOD:

1. Add all the required ingredients to a blender.
2. Blend for 2 minutes.
3. Transfer the shake to a large cup.
4. Stir and enjoy!

STORAGE INFORMATION:

Storage	Temperature	Expiration date	Preparation
Ziploc bag	Fridge at 38 – 40°F or 3°C	2-3 days after preparation	
Ziploc bag	Freezer at -1°F or -20°C	30 days after preparation	

Strawberries, orange, and protein—this smoothie is simple and great as a post-workout shake.

5. Powerhouse Protein Shake

Nutrition Information
(per serving)
- Calories: 257 kcal
- Carbs: 30 g.
- Fat: 3.5 g.
- Protein: 26.3 g.
- Fiber: 5.1 g.
- Sugar: 21.6 g.

INGREDIENTS:
- 2 green apples (peeled, cored, and chopped)
- 1 cup pineapple chunks (fresh or frozen)
- 1 cup kale (fresh, chopped)
- 1 cup spinach (drained and rinsed)
- 1 tsp. spirulina
- 1 cup coconut water (alternatively use 3-4 ice cubes)
- 2 scoops of vegan protein powder (unflavored)

Total number of ingredients: 7

METHOD:
1. Add all the required ingredients to a blender.
2. Blend for 2 minutes.
3. Transfer to a large cup or shaker.
4. Enjoy!

STORAGE INFORMATION:

Storage	Temperature	Expiration date	Preparation
Ziploc bag	Fridge at 38 – 40°F or 3°C	2-3 days after preparation	
Ziploc bag	Freezer at -1°F or -20°C	30 days after preparation	

This shake is full of antioxidant power and is ideal as a rest day / cleansing smoothie!

6. Avocado-Chia Protein Shake

Serves: 2 | Prep Time: ~10 min |

Nutrition Information
(per serving)
- Calories: 379 kcal
- Carbs: 16.6 g.
- Fat: 21.4 g.
- Protein: 30.1 g.
- Fiber: 9.8 g.
- Sugar: 2.8 g.

INGREDIENTS:

- ¼ cup dry chia seeds
- 1 cup coconut milk
- ½ avocado (pitted, peeled)
- 1½ tbsp. peanut butter
- 2 scoops of vegan protein powder
  (chocolate flavor)
- 1 cup water
- 3 ice cubes (optional)
- 1-2 tsp. cacao powder (optional)

Total number of ingredients: 8

METHOD:

1. Soak the chia seeds according the "Soaking and sprouting chia, hemp and flaxseeds" on page 10. Drain any excess water.
2. Add all the required, and if desired, optional ingredients to a blender. When using ice cubes, the water can be left out.
3. Blend for 2 minutes.
4. Transfer the shake to a large cup or shaker.
5. Top with some additional cacao powder.
6. Serve and enjoy!

STORAGE INFORMATION:

Storage	Temperature	Expiration date	Preparation
Ziploc bag	Fridge at 38 – 40°F or 3°C	2-3 days after preparation	
Ziploc bag	Freezer at -1°F or -20°C	30 days after preparation	

A healthy, protein-rich "premium shake" full of nutrients, this shake is also low in carbohydrates.

7. Almond & Protein Shake

Nutrition Information
(per serving)
- Calories: 340 kcal
- Carbs: 15.2 g.
- Fat: 17 g.
- Protein: 31.6 g.
- Fiber: 1.7 g.
- Sugar: 6.9 g.

INGREDIENTS:

- 1½ cups soy milk
- 3 tbsp. almonds
- 1 tsp. maple syrup
- 1 tbsp. coconut oil
- 2 scoops of vegan protein powder
  (chocolate or vanilla flavor)
- 2-4 ice cubes
- 1 tsp. cocoa powder (optional)

Total number of ingredients: 7

METHOD:

1. Add all the required ingredients, and if desired, the optional cocoa powder, to a blender.
2. Blend for 2 minutes.
3. Transfer the shake to a large cup or shaker.
4. Enjoy!

STORAGE INFORMATION:

Storage	Temperature	Expiration date	Preparation
Ziploc bag	Fridge at 38 – 40°F or 3°C	2-3 days after preparation	
Ziploc bag	Freezer at -1°F or -20°C	30 days after preparation	

All in one drink… almonds, soy, and plant-based protein.

Add more coconut oil for a higher fat count.

8. Oatmeal Protein Mix

- Calories: 298 kcal
- Carbs: 24.7 g.
- Fat: 9 g.
- Protein: 29.3 g.
- Fiber: 3.9 g.
- Sugar: 2.2 g.

INGREDIENTS:

- 1 cup dry oatmeal
- 3 scoops of vegan protein powder (chocolate or vanilla flavor)
- ½ tsp. cinnamon
- ½ tsp. maple syrup
- ¼ cup almonds
- 1 cup oat milk (alternatively use almond milk)
- 2 ice cubes
- 2 tbsp. peanut butter (optional)

Total number of ingredients: 8

METHOD:

1. Add the required ingredients, including the optional peanut butter if desired, to a blender.
2. Blend for 2 minutes.
3. Transfer to a large cup or shaker and enjoy!

STORAGE INFORMATION:

Storage	Temperature	Expiration date	Preparation
Ziploc bag	Fridge at 38 – 40°F or 3°C	2-3 days after preparation	
Ziploc bag	Freezer at -1°F or -20°C	30 days after preparation	

This shake has it all: fats, protein, and carbs in a tasty drink… perfect for breakfast or a quick meal!

9. Almond Explosion

Nutrition Information
(per serving)
- Calories: 355 kcal
- Carbs: 29.5 g.
- Fat: 15 g.
- Protein: 25.4 g.
- Fiber: 4.3 g.
- Sugar: 16.8 g.

INGREDIENTS:
- 1½ cups almond milk (unsweet-ened or homemade)
- ½ cup dry oatmeal
- ½ cup raisins
- ½ cup almonds
- ½ cup water
- 3 tbsp. peanut butter
- 3 scoops of vegan protein powder (vanilla flavor)
- ½ tsp. cinnamon (optional)
- 2 ice cubes (optional)

Total number of ingredients: 9

METHOD:
1. Add all the required ingredients, including the optional cinnamon if desired, to a blender.
2. Blend for 2 minutes.
3. Transfer the shake to a large cup.
4. Microwave the shake for a hot treat, or, add in the ice cubes and drink the shake with a straw.
5. Stir and enjoy!

STORAGE INFORMATION:

Storage	Temperature	Expiration date	Preparation
Ziploc bag	Fridge at 38 – 40°F or 3°C	2-3 days after preparation	
Ziploc bag	Freezer at -1°F or -20°C	30 days after preparation	

An explosion of almonds and protein… it's hard not to love this shake.

10. Protein Pancakes

Serves: 4| Prep Time: ~35 min |

Nutrition Information
(per serving)
- Calories: 113 kcal.
- Carbs: 5.3g.
- Fat: 7.6g.
- Protein: 7.8g.
- Fiber: 3.8g.
- Sugar: 0.7g.

INGREDIENTS:

- 1 scoop vegan protein powder
- ¼ cup almond flour
- 1 tbsp. glucomannan powder
- 1½ cup water
- 1 tbsp. flaxseed oil
- 2 tbsp. olive oil
- 1 tsp. vanilla extract
- 1 tsp. baking powder

Total number of ingredients: 8

METHOD:

1. Soak the glucomannan powder in ½ cup of water for a couple of minutes.
2. Combine the vegan protein powder, baking powder and almond flour in a medium bowl and set the dry ingredients aside.
3. Mix the vanilla extract and flaxseed oil with the soaked glucomannan.
4. Put a non-stick pan on the stove over medium heat and add two tablespoons olive oil.
5. Slowly stir the remaining cup of water into the dry flour mixture and combine thoroughly.
6. Add the glucomannan mixture and stir well.
7. Add a heap of batter to the pan and spread it out into a ¼ inch thick pancake.
8. Bake for 5 minutes on each side and repeat this for all the pancakes.
9. Enjoy or store!

STORAGE INFORMATION:

Storage	Temperature	Expiration date	Preparation
Ziploc bag	Fridge at 38 – 40°F or 3°C	3-4 days after preparation	Reheat in microwave.
Ziploc bag	Freezer at -1°F or -20°C	60 days after preparation	Thaw at room temperature. Reheat in microwave.

Tip: smaller pancakes are easier to store!

HIGH PROTEIN SALADS

1. Lentil, Lemon & Mushroom Salad

Serves: 2 | Prep Time: ~10 min |

Nutrition Information
(per serving)
- Calories: 262 kcal
- Carbs: 28.1 g.
- Fat: 9.6 g.
- Protein: 15.8 g.
- Fiber: 14.8 g.
- Sugar: 9.3 g.

INGREDIENTS:
- ½ cup dry lentils of choice
- 2 cups vegetable broth (page 17)
- 3 cups mushrooms (thickly sliced)
- 1 cup sweet or purple onion (chopped)
- 4 tsp. extra virgin olive oil
- 2 tbsp. garlic powder (or 3 garlic cloves, minced)
- ¼ tsp. chili flakes
- 1 tbsp. lemon juice
- 2 tbsp. cilantro (chopped)
- ½ cup arugula
- Salt and pepper to taste

Total number of ingredients: 12

METHOD:
1. Sprout the lentils according the "Sprouting" on page 9. (Don't cook them).
2. Place the vegetable stock in a deep saucepan and bring it to a boil.
3. Add the lentils to the boiling broth, cover the pan, and cook for about 5 minutes over low heat until the lentils are a bit tender.
4. Remove the pan from heat and drain the excess water.
5. Put a frying pan over high heat and add 2 tablespoons of olive oil.
6. Add the onions, garlic, and chili flakes, and cook until the onions are almost translucent, around 5 to 10 minutes while stirring.
7. Add the mushrooms to the frying pan and mix in thoroughly. Continue cooking until the onions are completely translucent and the mushrooms have softened; remove the pan from the heat.
8. Mix the lentils, onions, mushrooms, and garlic in a large bowl.
9. Add the lemon juice and the remaining olive oil. Toss or stir to combine everything thoroughly.
10. Serve the mushroom/onion mixture over some arugala in bowl, adding salt and pepper to taste, or, store and enjoy later!

STORAGE INFORMATION:

Storage	Temperature	Expiration date	Preparation
Airtight container M/L	Fridge at 38 – 40°F or 3°C	3-4 days after preparation	
Airtight container M/L	Freezer at -1°F or -20°C	60 days after preparation	Thaw at room temperature; Reheat in pot or microwave

Note: Add a handful of spinach or other leafy greens for a heartier salad.

Tip: Use thickly sliced button or swiss brown mushrooms for the best results.

2. Lentil Radish Salad

Serves: 3 | Prep Time: ~15 min |

Nutrition Information
(per serving)
- Calories: 247 kcal
- Carbs: 25.3 g.
- Fat: 10.7 g.
- Protein: 12.4 g.
- Fiber: 7.9 g.
- Sugar: 8.1 g.

INGREDIENTS:

Dressing:
- 1 tbsp. extra virgin olive oil
- 1 tbsp. lemon juice
- 1 tbsp. maple syrup (alternatively, use another sweetener)
- 1 tbsp. water
- ½ tbsp. sesame oil
- 1 tbsp. miso paste (yellow or white)
- ¼ tsp. salt
- Pepper to taste

Salad:
- ½ cup dry chickpeas
- ¼ cup dry green or brown lentils
- 1 14-oz. pack of silken tofu
- 5 cups mixed greens (fresh or frozen)
- 2 radishes (sliced thinly)
- ½ cup cherry tomatoes, halved
- ¼ cup roasted sesame seeds (optional)

Total number of ingredients: 15

METHOD:
1. Prepare the chickpeas according to the "Soaking and sprouting chia, hemp and flaxseeds" on page 10.
2. Prepare the lentils according to the "Sprouting" on page 9.
3. Put all the ingredients for the dressing in a blender or food processor. Mix on low until smooth, while adding water until it reaches the desired consistency.
4. Add salt, pepper (to taste), and optionally more water to the dressing and set aside.
5. Cut the tofu into bite-sized cubes.
6. Combine the mixed greens, tofu, lentils, chickpeas, radishes, and tomatoes in a large bowl.
7. Add the dressing and mix everything until it is coated evenly.
8. Top with the optional roasted sesame seeds, if desired.
9. Refrigerate before serving and enjoy, or, store for later!

STORAGE INFORMATION:

Storage	Temperature	Expiration date	Preparation
Airtight container M/L	Fridge at 38 – 40°F or 3°C	4-5 days after preparation	
Airtight container M/L	Freezer at -1°F or -20°C	60 days after preparation	Thaw at room temperature

Note: Extra sunflower seeds, roasted sesame seeds, or black-eyed beans taste great on this salad and add more nutrients!

Tip: If you don't have miso paste, you can replace it with the same amount of tahini.

3. Shaved Brussel Sprout Salad

Serves: 4 | Prep Time: ~25 min |

Nutrition Information
(per serving)

- Calories: 396 kcal
- Carbs: 45.3 g.
- Fat: 18.7 g.
- Protein: 11.5 g.
- Fiber: 14.1 g.
- Sugar: 18.4 g.

INGREDIENTS:

Dressing:

- 1 tbsp. brown mustard
- 1 tbsp. maple syrup
- 2 tbsp. apple cider vinegar
- 2 tbsp. extra virgin olive oil
- ½ tbsp. garlic (minced)

Salad:

- ½ cup dry red kidney beans
- ¼ cup dry chickpeas
- 2 cups brussel sprouts
- 1 cup purple onion
- 1 small sour apple
- ½ cup slivered almonds (crushed)
- ½ cup walnuts (crushed)
- ½ cup cranberries (dried)
- Salt and pepper to taste

Total number of ingredients: 15

METHOD:

1. Prepare the beans according to the"Soaking and cooking time per bean or legume" on page 7.
2. Combine all dressing ingredients in a small bowl and stir well until combined.
3. Refrigerate the dressing for up to one hour before serving.
4. Use a grater, mandolin, or knife to thinly slice each brussel sprout. Repeat this with the apple and onion.
5. Take a large bowl to mix the chickpeas, beans, sprouts, apples, onions, cranberries, and nuts.
6. Drizzle the cold dressing and over the salad to coat.
7. Serve with salt and pepper to taste, or, store for later!

STORAGE INFORMATION:

Storage	Temperature	Expiration date	Preparation
Airtight container M/L	Fridge at 38 – 40°F or 3°C	4-5 days after preparation	
Airtight container M/L	Freezer at -1°F or -20°C	60 days after preparation	Thaw at room temperature

Note: Toasted almonds and walnuts taste great with the sour apples, especially Granny Smith apples.

Tip: Shred the brussel sprouts very thinly for the best salad flavor.

4. Colorful Protein Power Salad

Serves: 2 | Prep Time: ~20 min |

Nutrition Information
(per serving)
- Calories: 487 kcal.
- Carbs: 64.8 g.
- Fat: 15.5 g.
- Protein: 22.3 g.
- Fiber: 17.4 g.
- Sugar: 6 g.

INGREDIENTS:

- ½ cup dry quinoa
- 2 cups dry navy beans
- 1 green onion (chopped)
- 2 tsp. garlic (minced)
- 3 cups green or purple cabbage (chopped)
- 4 cups kale (chopped, fresh or frozen)
- 1 cup shredded carrot (chopped)
- 2 tbsp. extra virgin olive oil
- 1 tsp. lemon juice
- Salt and pepper to taste

Total number of ingredients: 11

METHOD:

1. Prepare the quinoa according to the "Quinoa" on page 13.
2. Prepare the beans according to the "Soaking and cooking time per bean or legume" on page 7.
3. Heat up 1 tablespoon of the olive oil in a frying pan over medium heat.
4. Add the chopped green onion, garlic, and cabbage, and sauté for 2-3 minutes.
5. Add the kale, the remaining 1 tablespoon of olive oil and salt. Lower the heat and cover until the greens have wilted, around 5 minutes. Remove the pan from the stove and set aside.
6. Take a large bowl and mix the remaining ingredients with the kale and cabbage mixture once it has cooled down. Add more salt and pepper to taste.
7. Mix until everything is distributed evenly.
8. Serve topped with a dressing, or, store for later!

STORAGE INFORMATION:

Storage	Temperature	Expiration date	Preparation
Airtight container M/L	Fridge at 38 – 40°F or 3°C	4-5 days after preparation	
Airtight container M/L	Freezer at -1°F or -20°C	60 days after preparation	Thaw at room temperature

Note: Add olive oil and apple cider vinegar for a simple dressing. It's a great compliment to all the flavors here!

Tip: Use purple cabbage if possible. The milder flavor tastes better raw compared to green cabbage.

5. Taco Tempeh Salad

Nutrition Information
(per serving)

- Calories: 441 kcal
- Carbs: 36.3 g.
- Fat: 23 g.
- Protein: 22,4 g.
- Fiber: 17.6 g.
- Sugar: 4.1 g.

INGREDIENTS:

- 1 cup dry black beans
- 1 8-oz. package tempeh
- 1 tbsp. lime or lemon juice
- 2 tbsp. extra virgin olive oil
- 1 tsp. maple syrup
- ½ tsp. chili powder
- ¼ tsp. cumin
- ¼ tsp. paprika
- 1 large bunch of kale (chopped, fresh or frozen)
- 1 large avocado (peeled, pitted, diced)
- ½ cup salsa (page 19)
- Salt and pepper to taste

Total number of ingredients: 13

METHOD:

1. Prepare the beans according to the "Soaking and cooking time per bean or legume" on page 7.
2. Cut the tempeh into ¼-inch cubes; then add the cut tempeh, lime or lemon juice, 1 tablespoon of olive oil, maple syrup, chili powder, cumin, and paprika to a bowl.
3. Stir well and let the tempeh marinate in the fridge for at least 1 hour, up to 12 hours.
4. Heat the remaining 1 tablespoon of olive oil in a frying pan over medium heat.
5. Add the marinated tempeh mixture and cook until brown and crispy on both sides, around 10 minutes.
6. Put the chopped kale in a bowl with the cooked beans and prepared tempeh.
7. Store, or serve the salad immediately, topped with salsa, avocado, and salt and pepper to taste.

STORAGE INFORMATION:

Storage	Temperature	Expiration date	Preparation
Airtight container M/L	Fridge at 38 – 40°F or 3°C	3-4 days after preparation	
Airtight container M/L	Freezer at -1°F or -20°C	60 days after preparation	Thaw at room temperature

Note: You can also serve this salad with tortilla strips and vegan cheese on top.

Tip: Marinate the tempeh longer for more flavor.

STAPLE FOOD LUNCHES

1. Sweet Potato Chickpea Mingle

Serves: 2 | Prep Time: ~30 min |

Nutrition Information
(per serving)

- Calories: 379 kcal.
- Carbs: 33.4g.
- Fat: 20.2g.
- Protein 16g.
- Fiber: 27.8g.
- Sugar: 8.4g.

INGREDIENTS:

- 1 cup dry chickpeas
- 1 sweet potato (large, cubed)
- ½ tsp. ground cumin
- 1 tbsp. fresh ginger (minced)
- 1 tsp. spicy paprika powder
- Salt and pepper to taste
- 2 tbsp. water
- 2 tbsp. coconut oil
- 1 garlic clove (minced)
- 5 tbsp. baba ganoush (page 20)
- 1 tsp. tabasco sauce

Total number of ingredients: 11

METHOD:

1. Preheat oven to 400°F or 200°C.
2. Prepare the chickpeas according to the "Soaking and sprouting chia, hemp and flaxseeds" on page 10.
3. Take a baking sheet and grease it with 1 tablespoon of coconut oil.
4. Roast the sweet potato cubes in the oven for about 20 minutes and check them every five minutes. Use a fork to see if the cubes are softened. Turn the potato cubes to roast evenly. Set aside after roasting.
5. Place the cumin, fresh ginger, paprika powder, salt, pepper and water in a medium-sized bowl.
6. Stir well and add more spices to taste.
7. Take a large skillet and grease it with 1 tablespoon of coconut oil.
8. Put it on low heat and add the cooked chickpeas along with the minced garlic.
9. Carefully mash the mixture with a fork.
10. Cook for 4 minutes and add salt and pepper to taste.
11. Combine the mixture with the baba ganoush and spice mixture.
12. Stir well.
13. Top the mixture with tabasco sauce and enjoy!
14. Serve the chickpea mingled with the roasted potatoes
15. Enjoy or store the ingredients separately.

STORAGE INFORMATION:

Storage	Temperature	Expiration date	Preparation
2 compartment airtight container M/L	Fridge at 38 – 40°F or 3°C	4-5 days after preparation	Reheat in pot or microwave.
2 compartment airtight container M/L	Freezer at -1°F or -20°C	30 days after preparation	Thaw at room temperature. Reheat in pot or microwave.

Note: serve the dish with extra baba ganoush on the side. Use multiple compartment or separate containers to store the potatoes and chickpea mingle.

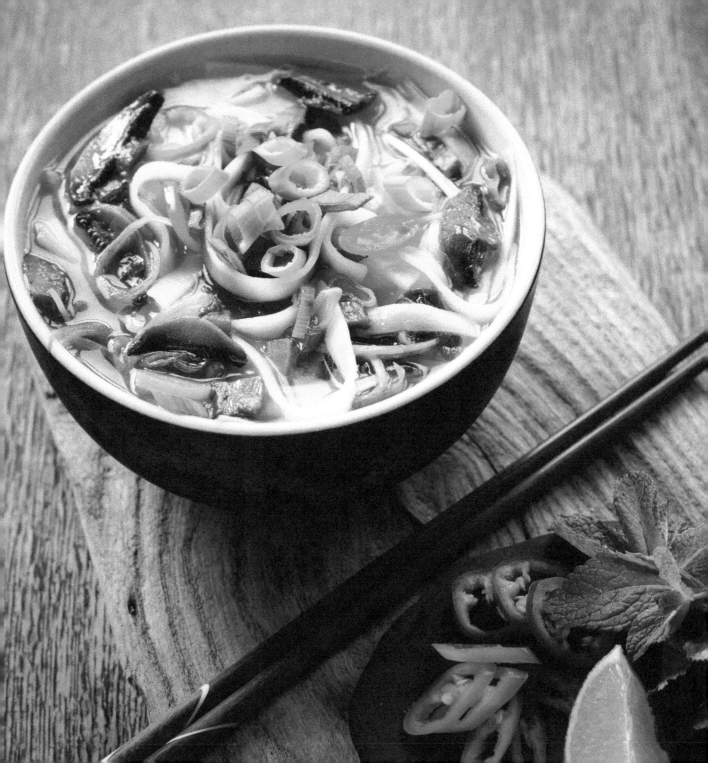

2. Vegan Mushroom Pho

Serves: 3 | Prep Time: ~10 min |

Nutrition Information
(per serving)
- Calories: 383 kcal
- Carbs: 57.3 g.
- Fat: 9.1 g.
- Protein: 17.8 g.
- Fiber: 9.4 g.
- Sugar: 3 g.

INGREDIENTS:
- 1 14-oz. block firm tofu (drained)
- 6 cups vegetable broth (page 17)
- 3 green onions (thinly sliced)
- 1 tsp. or ½-inch minced ginger
- 1 tsp. olive oil
- 3 cups mushrooms (sliced)
- 2 tbsp. hoisin sauce
- 1 tsp. sesame oil
- 2 cups gluten-free rice noodles
- 1 cup raw bean sprouts
- 1 cup matchstick carrots
- 1 cup bok choy (chopped, optional)
- 1 cup cabbage (chopped, optional)
- Salt and pepper to taste

Total number of ingredients: 15

METHOD:
1. Cut the tofu into ¼-inch cubes and set it aside.
2. Take a deep saucepan and heat the vegetable broth, green onions, and ginger over medium high heat.
3. Boil for 1 minute before reducing the heat to low; then cover the saucepan with a lid and let it simmer for 20 minutes.
4. Take another frying pan and heat the olive oil in it over medium-high heat.
5. Add the sliced mushrooms to the frying pan and cook until they are tender, for about 5 minutes.
6. Add the tofu, hoisin sauce, and sesame oil to the mushrooms.
7. Heat until the sauce thickens in about around 5 minutes and remove the frying pan from the heat.
8. Prepare the gluten-free rice noodles according to the package instructions.
9. Top the rice noodles with a scoop of the tofu mushroom mixture, a generous amount of broth, and the bean sprouts.
10. Add the carrots, and optional cabbage and/or bok choy (if desired), right before serving.
11. Top with salt and pepper to taste and enjoy, or, store ingredients separately!

STORAGE INFORMATION:

Storage	Temperature	Expiration date	Preparation
3-compartment airtight container M/L	Fridge at 38 – 40°F or 3°C	4-5 days after preparation	Reheat on stove or in microwave
3-compartment airtight container M/L	Freezer at -1°F or -20°C	60 days after preparation	Thaw at room temperature; Reheat in a pot or in the microwave

Note: For authentic pho flavors, add lime juice, cilantro, and basil as a garnish. For a spicier pho, add sliced jalapeños or sriracha!

Tip: Use low-sodium hoisin and broth to reduce salt intake. Store the noodles, tofu mushroom mixture, and broth separately.

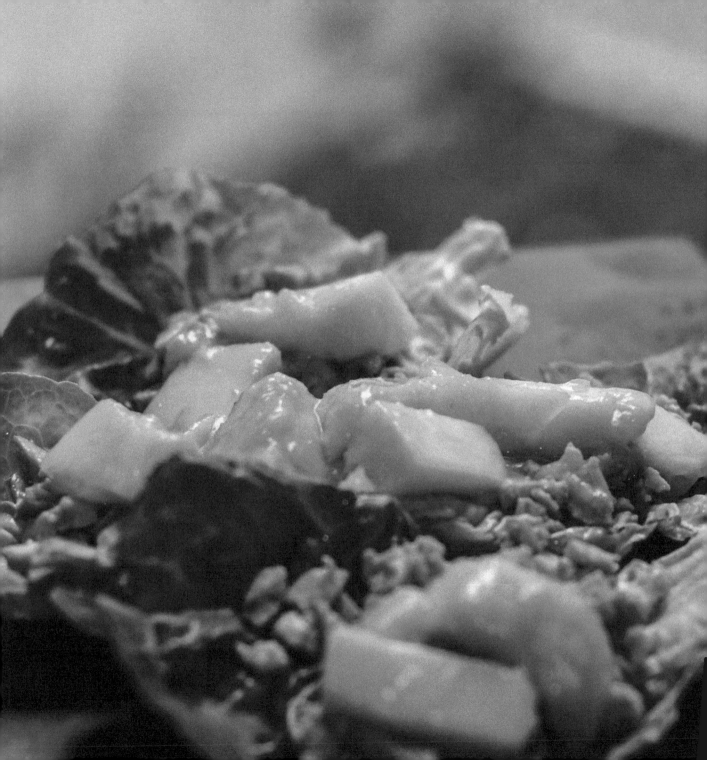

3. Mango-Tempeh Wraps

Nutrition Information
(per serving)

- Calories: 259 kcal
- Carbs: 31.3 g.
- Fat: 7.8 g.
- Protein: 15.7 g.
- Fiber: 9.7 g.
- Sugar: 16 g.

INGREDIENTS:

- 2 8-oz. blocks tempeh (drained, crumbled)
- 1 tbsp. coconut oil
- 6 large lettuce leaves
- 2 medium ripe mangoes (peeled, diced)
- ¼ cup sweet chili sauce
- 1 tbsp. hoisin sauce
- 1 tbsp. garlic powder
- ¼ tsp. lime juice
- ¼ tsp. salt

Total number of ingredients: 9

METHOD:

1. Heat the coconut oil in a large skillet over medium heat.
2. Cook the tempeh crumbles until browned, stirring constantly, for about 4 minutes and turn the heat down to low.
3. Add the hoisin, garlic, salt, and lime juice; heat for an additional 2 minutes and set aside.
4. Cut the mangoes into ¼-inch cubes. Pour the sweet chili sauce into a small bowl and mix it with the mango cubes.
5. Scoop the cooked tempeh and divide it eveny between the lettuce leaves, using the leaves as wraps.
6. Top the wraps with the chunks of mango and a bit of lime juice, and close the wraps.
7. Serve, share, or store!

STORAGE INFORMATION:

Storage	Temperature	Expiration date	Preparation
Airtight container M/L or Ziploc bag	Fridge at 38 – 40°F or 3°C	4-5 days after preparation	Eat chilled or reheat 10 seconds in the microwave
Airtight container M/L or Ziploc bag	Freezer at -1°F or -20°C	60 days after preparation	Thaw at room temperature; Eat chilled or reheat 10 seconds in the microwave

Note: Store the wraps already prepared, or, use multiple containers for the separate ingredients (tempeh, mangoes, and lettuce leaves).

4. Creamy Squash Pizza

Serves: 4 | Prep Time: ~25 min |

Nutrition Information
(per serving)
- Calories: 401 kcal
- Carbs: 62.5 g.
- Fat: 8.6 g.
- Protein: 18.4 g.
- Fiber: 15.2 g.
- Sugar: 8.8 g.

INGREDIENTS:

Sauce:
- 3 cups butternut squash (cubed, fresh or frozen)
- 2 tbsp. minced garlic
- 1 tbsp. olive oil
- 1 tsp. red pepper flakes
- 1 tsp. cumin
- 1 tsp. paprika
- 1 tsp. oregano

Crust:
- 2 cups dry French green lentils
- 2 cups water
- 2 tbsp. minced garlic
- 1 tbsp. Italian seasoning
- 1 tsp. onion powder

Toppings:
- 1 tbsp. olive oil
- 1 medium green bell pepper (pitted, diced)
- 1 small head of broccoli (diced)
- 1 medium red bell pepper (pitted, diced)
- 1 small purple onion (diced)

Total number of ingredients: 15

METHOD:

1. Preheat the oven to 350°F / 175°C.
2. Prepare the French green lentils according to the "Soaking and sprouting chia, hemp and flaxseeds" on page 10.
3. Add all the sauce ingredients to a food processor or blender, and blend on low until everything has mixed and the sauce looks creamy. Set the sauce aside in a small bowl.
4. Clean the food processor or blender; then add all the ingredients for the crust and pulse on high speed until a dough-like batter has formed.
5. Heat a large deep-dish pan over medium-low heat and lightly grease it with 1 tablespoon of olive oil.
6. Press the crust dough into the skillet until it resembles a round pizza crust and cook until the crust is golden brown—about 5-6 minutes on each side.
7. Put the crust on a baking tray covered with parchment paper.
8. Coat the topside of the crust with the sauce using a spoon, and evenly distribute the toppings across the pizza.
9. Bake the pizza in the oven until the vegetables are tender and browned, for about 15 minutes.
10. Slice into 4 equal pieces and serve, or store.

STORAGE INFORMATION:

Storage	Temperature	Expiration date	Preparation
Airtight container S/M or Ziploc bag	Fridge at 38 – 40°F or 3°C	4-5 days after preparation	Reheat in the microwave
Airtight container S/M or Ziploc bag	Freezer at -1°F or -20°C	60 days after preparation	Thaw at room temperature. Reheat in the microwave

Note: Top this pizza with extra toppings or other vegetables.

Tip: Use a large skillet and press the crust out as flatly as possible. This way, the crust cooks quicker.

5. Lasagna Fungo

Nutrition Information
(per serving)
- Calories: 292 kcal
- Carbs: 38 g.
- Fat: 9.2 g.
- Protein:14.2 g.
- Fiber: 6.3 g.
- Sugar: 4.9 g.

INGREDIENTS:

- 10 lasagna noodles or sheets
- 2 cups matchstick carrots
- 1 cup mushrooms (sliced)
- 2 cups raw kale
- 1 14-oz. package extra firm tofu (drained)
- 1 cup hummus (pre-made or (page 23))
- ½ cup nutritional yeast
- 2 tbsp. Italian seasoning
- 1 tbsp. garlic powder (or fresh, minced)
- 1 tbsp. olive oil
- 4 cups marinara sauce (page 21)
- 1 tsp. salt

Total number of ingredients: 12

METHOD:

1. Preheat the oven to 400°F / 200°C.
2. Cook the lasagna noodles or sheets according to according to the package instructions.
3. Take a large frying pan, put it over medium heat, and add the olive oil.
4. Throw in the carrots, mushrooms, and ½ teaspoon salt; cook for 5 minutes.
5. Add the kale, sauté for another 3 minutes, and remove the pan from the heat.
6. Take a large bowl, crumble in the tofu, and set the bowl aside for now.
7. Take another bowl, add the hummus, nutritional yeast, Italian seasoning, garlic, and ½ teaspoon salt; mix everything together.
8. Coat the bottom of an 8x8 baking dish with 1 cup of the marinara sauce.
9. Cover the sauce with a couple of the noodles or sheets, and top these with the tofu crumbles.
10. Add a layer of the vegetables on top of the tofu.
11. Continue to build up the lasagna by stacking layers of marinara sauce, noodles or sheets, tofu, and vegetables, and top it off with a cup of marinara sauce.
12. Cover the lasagna with aluminum foil, and bake in the oven for 20-25 minutes.
13. Remove the foil and put back in the oven for an additional 5 minutes.
14. Allow the lasagna to sit for 10 minutes before serving, or store for another day!

STORAGE INFORMATION:

Storage	Temperature	Expiration date	Preparation
Airtight container M/L	Fridge at 38 – 40°F or 3°C	4-5 days after preparation	Reheat in pot or microwave
Airtight container M/L	Freezer at -1°F or -20°C	60 days after preparation	Thaw at room temperature; Reheat in pot or microwave

Note: Top this lasagna with some vegan cheese before the last 5 minutes of baking for an ooey, gooey dish.

Tip: You can replace the lasagna noodles or sheets with sliced eggplant for a lower carb count and different flavor!

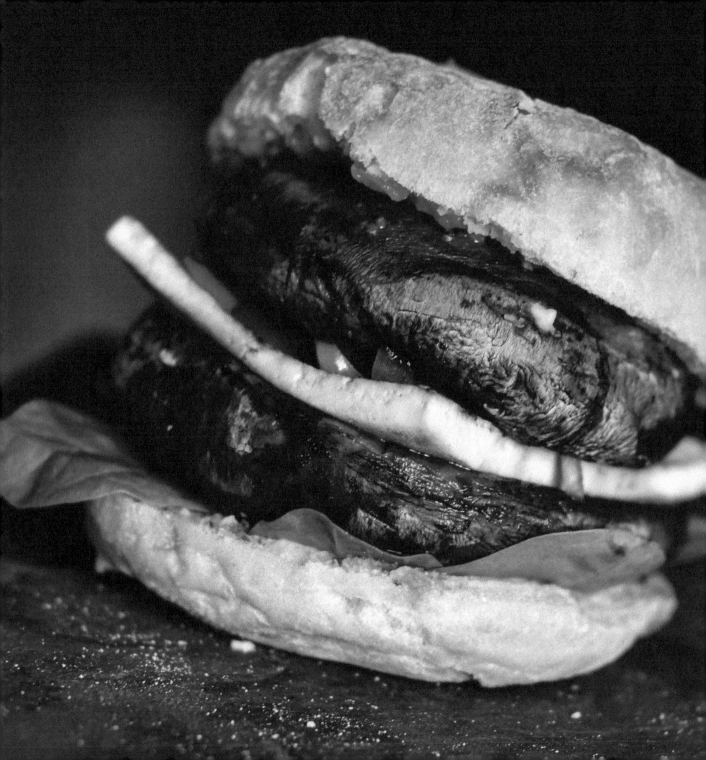

6. Stacked N' Spicy Portobello Burgers

Serves: 2 | Prep Time: ~20 min |

Nutrition Information (per serving without bun)

- Calories: 421 kcal
- Carbs: 48.9 g.
- Fat: 16 g.
- Protein: 20.5 g.
- Fiber: 9.8 g.
- Sugar: 10.6 g.

INGREDIENTS:

- 1 8-oz. block firm tofu (drained)
- 1 tbsp. extra virgin olive oil
- 4 large portobello mushroom caps (stems removed)
- 1 large onion (diced)
- ½ green bell pepper (pitted, diced)
- ½ red bell pepper (pitted, diced)
- 3 cups spinach (fresh, rinsed, dried)
- 2 whole wheat vegan buns
- 4 tbsp. hummus (pre-made or (page 23))
- ¼ cup salsa (page 19)
- 1 tbsp. taco seasoning
- ½ tsp. paprika
- ¼ tsp. chili powder
- Salt to taste

Total number of ingredients: 14

METHOD:

1. Cut the tofu into 4 large slices and set aside.
2. Heat the olive oil in a large skillet over medium-high heat.
3. Add the mushroom caps and flip them over after 4 minutes of cooking.
4. Sprinkle the caps with the taco seasoning, paprika, chili powder, and salt.
5. Flip again after 4 minutes, allowing them to cook until they have halved in size. Remove the caps from the skillet and set aside.
6. Add the tofu slices to the previously used skillet and cook them on both sides until slightly brown; set them aside.
7. Add the diced onions and bell peppers to the skillet. Stir frequently and cook the vegetables until browned, for 10-12 minutes.
8. Turn the heat down to low and add the mushrooms back to the skillet, and reheat for 2 more minutes.
9. Spread hummus on one side of each bun, and the salsa on the other half.
10. Top the hummus with a handful of spinach and serve with two mushroom caps, tofu squares, and top with a heaping scoop of vegetables with more salt to taste.
11. Enjoy the portobello burgers right away, or store and serve later!

STORAGE INFORMATION:

Storage	Temperature	Expiration date	Preparation
Airtight container M/L and Ziploc bag	Fridge at 38 – 40°F or 3°C	2-3 days after preparation	
Airtight container M/L and Ziploc bag	Freezer at -1°F or -20°C	60 days after preparation	Thaw at room temperature

Note: A thick slice of juicy tomato will really make these burgers pop! For storing, use a container for all the heated ingredients and a Ziploc bag for the buns or wraps.

Tip: Press down on the Portobello caps with a wooden spoon to remove the excess water faster.

7. Spicy Black Bean Soup & Tortilla Chips

Serves: 3 | Prep Time: ~15 min |

Nutrition Information
(per serving)
- Calories: 829 kcal.
- Carbs: 110g.
- Fat: 34g.
- Protein: 20.8g.
- Fiber: 16.8g.
- Sugar: 13g.

INGREDIENTS:

- 1 bag (300g) tortilla chips
- 2 cups dry black beans
- 2 tbsp. olive oil
- 2 yellow onions (large, chopped)
- 3 celery ribs (finely chopped)
- 2 carrots (medium, peeled and sliced)
- 4 cups vegetable broth (page 17)
- 6 garlic cloves (minced)
- 2 tbsp. ground cumin
- ½ tsp. red pepper flakes
- 3 tbsp. fresh lime juice
- 1 tsp. of sherry vinegar
- Sea salt and ground black pepper to taste
- 2 tsp. of lime juice

Total number of ingredients: 14

METHOD:

1. Prepare the black beans according to the "Soaking and cooking time per bean or legume" on page 7.
2. Place a large soup pot on medium heat.
3. Add the olive oil, onions, celery and carrots to the pot.
4. Add a pinch of salt and blend in the vegetable broth.
5. Stir occasionally and cook the soup for about 10 minutes.
6. Add the garlic, cumin and pepper flakes.
7. Add the beans to the soup.
8. Lower the heat and let the soup simmer for about 20 minutes, covered.
9. Blend the soup in a blender until smooth (depending on the size of the blender, in 2-3 parts).
10. Return the blended soup to the soup pot.
11. Stir in the lime juice, sherry vinegar and pepper.
12. Add more spices like salt and pepper to taste.
13. Serve in a bowl with 100 g of tortilla chips on the side.
14. Enjoy or store!

STORAGE INFORMATION:

Storage	Temperature	Expiration date	Preparation
Airtight container M/L & Ziploc bag S	Fridge at 38 – 40°F or 3°C	4-5 days after preparation	Reheat the soup in pot or microwave
Airtight container M/L & Ziploc bag S	Freezer at -1°F or -20°C	60 days after preparation	Thaw at room temperature. Reheat the soup in pot or microwave

Note: store the tortilla chips in separate Ziploc bags per portion to prevent deviant portion sizes. Alternatively keep the chips in the original package.

8. Stuffed Sweet Potatoes

Nutrition Information
(per serving)
- Calories: 498 kcal
- Carbs: 55.7 g.
- Fat: 17.1 g.
- Protein: 20.7 g.
- Fiber: 19.1 g.
- Sugar: 10.6 g.

INGREDIENTS:
- ½ cup dry black beans
- 3 sweet potatoes (small or medium)
- 2 tbsp. olive oil
- 1 large red bell pepper (pitted, chopped)
- 1 large green bell pepper (pitted, chopped)
- 1 small sweet yellow onion (chopped)
- 2 tbsp. garlic (minced or powdered)
- 1 8-oz. package tempeh (diced into ¼" cubes)
- ½ cup marinara sauce (page 21)
- ½ cup water
- 1 tbsp. chili powder
- 1 tsp. parsley
- ½ tsp. cayenne
- Salt and pepper to taste

Total number of ingredients: 15

METHOD:
1. Preheat the oven to 400°F / 200°C.
2. Prepare the black beans according to the "Soaking and cooking time per bean or legume" on page 7.
3. Using a fork, poke several holes in the skins of the sweet potatoes.
4. Wrap the sweet potatoes tightly with aluminum foil and place them in the oven until soft and tender, or for approximately 45 minutes.
5. Meanwhile, heat the olive oil in a deep pan over medium-high heat. Add the onions, bell peppers, and garlic; cook until the onions are tender, for about 10 minutes.
6. Add the water, together with the cooked beans, marinara sauce, chili powder, parsley, and cayenne. Bring the mixture to a boil and then lower the heat to medium or low. Allow the mixture to simmer until the liquid has thickened, for about 15 minutes.
7. Add the diced tempeh cubes and heat until warmed, around 1 minute.
8. Blend in salt and pepper to taste.
9. When the potatoes are done baking, remove them from the oven. Cut a slit across the top of each one, but do not split the potatoes all the way in half.
10. Top each potato with a scoop of the beans, vegetables, and tempeh mixture. Place the filled potatoes back in the hot oven for about 5 minutes.
11. Serve after cooling for a few minutes, or, store for another day!

STORAGE INFORMATION:

Storage	Temperature	Expiration date	Preparation
2-compartment airtight container M/L	Fridge at 38 – 40°F or 3°C	4-5 days after preparation	Reheat in pot or microwave
2-compartment airtight container M/L	Freezer at -1°F or -20°C	60 days after preparation	Thaw at room temperature; Reheat in pot or microwave

Note: You can replace the sweet potatoes with bell peppers, squash, eggplants, and more! The possibilities are endless but note that the oven time may differ.

Tip: If the filling seems too thick, add a tablespoon of water. If it seems too runny, add a touch of cornstarch to thicken.

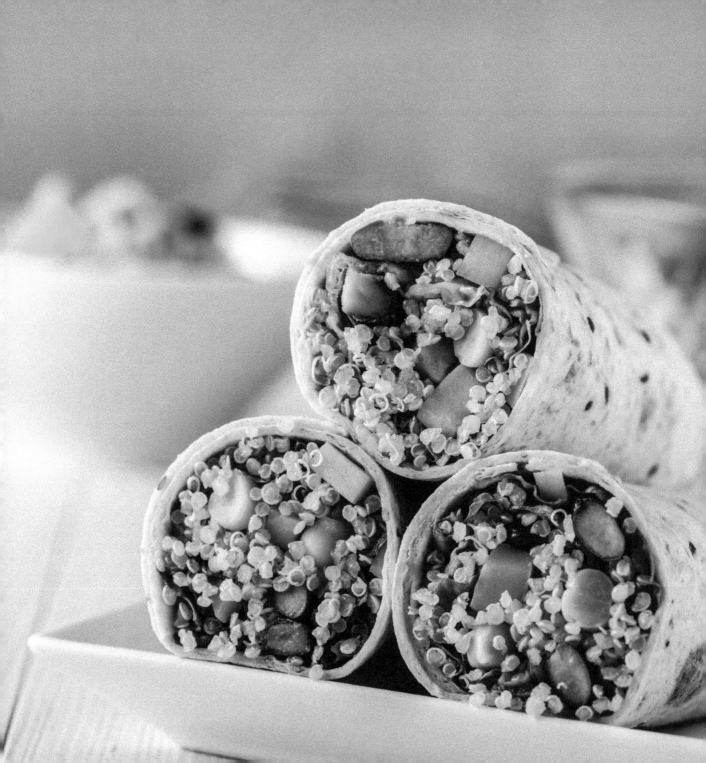

9. Black Bean and Quinoa Burrito

Nutrition Information
(per serving)
- Calories: 493 kcal.
- Carbs: 84g.
- Fat: 8.8g.
- Protein: 16.5g.
- Fiber: 14.5g.
- Sugar: 6.6g.

INGREDIENTS:
- 2 cups dry black beans
- ½ cup dry quinoa
- 2 tbsp. canola oil
- 2 onions (medium, diced)
- 5 cloves garlic (minced)
- 1 jalapeño (seeded, minced)
- 1 red bell pepper (large, diced)
- 1 zucchini (medium, diced)
- 1 (200g) can of sweet corn (drained)
- 1 large tomato (diced)
- 1 tbsp. cumin
- 1 tsp. sweet paprika powder
- 1 tsp. chili powder
- 1 tsp. salt
- ½ bunch of cilantro (chopped)
- 2 tsp. lemon juice
- 6 tortillas (large, whole wheat)

Total number of ingredients: 17

METHOD:
1. Prepare the black beans according to the "Soaking and cooking time per bean or legume" on page 7.
2. Prepare the quinoa according to the "Quinoa" on page 13.
3. Grease a large skillet with canola oil and put it on medium heat.
4. Sauté the onions for about 5 minutes until browned.
5. Add the garlic and jalapeños to the skillet and stir the ingredients for about 2 minutes.
6. Toss in the zucchini, jalapeño, red bell pepper, corn and tomato.
7. Cook the mixture for about 5 minutes while stirring.
8. Stir in the cooked beans, cumin, paprika powder, chili powder and add salt to the mix.
9. Add the cooked quinoa to the skillet. Stir everything before removing the skillet from the heat.
10. Put 4-5 tablespoons of the mixture on a tortilla and top it with fresh cilantro and lemon juice.
11. Wrap it tightly and enjoy right away or store the mixture and tortillas separately!

STORAGE INFORMATION:

Storage	Temperature	Expiration date	Preparation
Airtight container M/L and Ziploc bag	Fridge at 38 – 40°F or 3°C	3-4 days after preparation	Reheat in pot or microwave
Airtight container M/L and Ziploc bag	Freezer at -1°F or -20°C	60 days after preparation	Thaw at room temperature. Reheat in pot or microwave

Note: use a container and a Ziploc bag for the tortillas and black bean mixture. Keep the cilantro in the original package and take out a small portion on the day of consumption. Same goes for the lemon; alternatively, slice a lemon in 3-6 pieces and wrap these in foil.

10. Satay Tempeh with Cauliflower Rice

Serves: 4 | Prep Time: ~60 min |

Nutrition Information
(per serving)

- Calories: 531 kcal
- Carbs: 31.7 g.
- Fat: 33 g.
- Protein: 27.6 g.
- Fiber: 14.8 g.
- Sugar: 10.4 g.

INGREDIENTS:

Sauce:

- ¼ cup water
- 4 tbsp. peanut butter (page 24)
- 3 tbsp. low sodium soy sauce
- 2 tbsp. coconut sugar
- 1 garlic clove (minced)
- ½-inch ginger (minced)
- 2 tsp. rice vinegar
- 1 tsp. red pepper flakes

Main ingredients:

- 4 tbsp. olive oil
- 2 8-oz. packages tempeh (drained)
- 2 cups cauliflower rice
- 1 cup purple cabbage (diced)
- 1 tbsp. sesame oil
- 1 tsp. agave nectar

Total number of ingredients: 14

METHOD:

1. Take a large bowl, combine all the ingredients for the sauce, and then whisk until the mixture is smooth and any lumps have dissolved.
2. Cut the tempeh into ½-inchg cubes and put them into the sauce, stirring to make sure the cubes get coated thoroughly.
3. Place the bowl in the refrigerator to marinate the tempeh for up to 3 hours.
4. Before the tempeh is done marinating, preheat the oven to 400°F / 200°C.
5. Spread the tempeh out in a single layer on a baking sheet lined with parchment paper or lightly greased with olive oil.
6. Bake the marinated cubes until browned and crisp—about 15 minutes.
7. Heat the cauliflower rice in a saucepan with 2 tablespoons of olive oil over medium heat until it is warm.
8. Rinse the large bowl with water, and then mix the cabbage, sesame oil and agave together.
9. Serve a scoop of the cauliflower rice topped with the marinated cabbage and cooked tempeh on a plate or in a bowl and enjoy, or, store for later.

STORAGE INFORMATION:

Storage	Temperature	Expiration date	Preparation
3-compartment airtight container M/L	Fridge at 38 – 40°F or 3°C	4-5 days after preparation	Reheat in pot or microwave
3-compartment airtight container M/L	Freezer at -1°F or -20°C	60 days after preparation	Thaw at room temperature; Reheat in pot or microwave

Note: Sesame seeds make a great garnish! Store the cauliflower rice, cabbage, and tempeh in a 3-compartment container or separate containers.

Tip: Use a food processor to make rice from a head of fresh cauliflower.

11. Teriyaki Tofu Wraps

Serves: 3 | Prep Time: ~25 min |

Nutrition Information
(per serving)
- Calories: 259 kcal
- Carbs: 20.5 g.
- Fat: 15.4 g.
- Protein: 12.1 g.
- Fiber: 3.2 g.
- Sugar: 11.6 g.

INGREDIENTS:

- 1 14-oz. package extra firm tofu
  (drained)
- 1 small white onion (diced)
- ½ pineapple (peeled, cored)
- ¼ cup soy sauce
- 2 tbsp. sesame oil
- 1 garlic clove (minced, or ½ tsp.
  garlic powder)
- 1 tbsp. coconut sugar
- 3-6 large lettuce leaves
- 1 tbsp. roasted sesame seeds
- Salt and pepper to taste

Total number of ingredients: 11

METHOD:

1. Take a medium-sized bowl and mix the soy sauce, sesame oil, coconut sugar, and garlic.
2. Cut the tofu into ½-inch cubes, place them in the bowl, and transfer the bowl to the refrigerator to marinate, up to 3 hours.
3. Meanwhile, cut the pineapple into rings or cubes.
4. After the tofu is adequately marinated, place a large skillet over medium heat, and pour in the tofu with the remaining marinade, pineapple cubes, and diced onions; stir.
5. Add salt and pepper to taste, making sure to stir the ingredients frequently, and cook until the onions are soft and translucent—about 15 minutes.
6. Divide the mixture between the lettuce leaves and top with a sprinkle of roasted sesame seeds.
7. Serve right away, or, store the mixture and lettuce leaves separately.

STORAGE INFORMATION:

Storage	Temperature	Expiration date	Preparation
2-compartment airtight container M	Fridge at 38 – 40°F or 3°C	4-5 days after preparation	Reheat in pot or microwave
2-compartment airtight container M	Freezer at -1°F or -20°C	60 days after preparation	Thaw at room temperature; Reheat in pot or microwave

Note: Butter, Bibb and Iceberg lettuce leaves work best for these wraps.

Tip: Replace the soy sauce with tamari for a different taste and a gluten-free dish.

12. Tex-Mex Tofu & Beans

Serves: 4 | Prep Time: ~25 min |

Nutrition Information
(per serving)
- Calories: 315 kcal
- Carbs: 27.8 g.
- Fat: 17 g.
- Protein: 12.7 g.
- Fiber: 7.5 g.
- Sugar: 1.9 g.

INGREDIENTS:

- 1 cup dry black beans
- 1 cup dry brown rice
- 1 14-oz. package firm tofu
  (drained)
- 2 tbsp. olive oil
- 1 small purple onion (diced)
- 1 medium avocado (pitted, peeled)
- 1 garlic clove (minced)
- 1 tbsp. lime juice
- 2 tsp. cumin
- 2 tsp. paprika
- 1 tsp. chili powder
- Salt and pepper to taste

Total number of ingredients: 13

METHOD:

1. Prepare the black beans according to the "Soaking and cooking time per bean or legume" on page 7.
2. Prepare the brown rice according to the "Method for medium-grain rice:" on page 11.
3. Cut the tofu into ½-inch cubes.
4. Heat the olive oil in a large skillet over high heat. Add the diced onions and cook until soft, for about 5 minutes.
5. Add the tofu and cook an additional 2 minutes, flipping the cubes frequently.
6. Meanwhile, cut the avocado into thin slices and set aside.
7. Lower the heat to medium and mix in the garlic, cumin, and cooked black beans.
8. Stir until everything is incorporated thoroughly and cook for an additional 5 minutes.
9. Add the remaining spices and lime juice to the mixture in the skillet.
10. Mix thoroughly and remove the skillet from the heat.
11. Serve the Tex-Mex tofu and beans with a scoop of rice and garnish it with fresh avocado.
12. Enjoy immediately, or, store the rice, avocado, and tofu mixture separately!

STORAGE INFORMATION:

Storage	Temperature	Expiration date	Preparation
3-compartment airtight container M/L	Fridge at 38 – 40°F or 3°C	4-5 days after preparation	Reheat in pot or microwave
3-compartment airtight container M/L	Freezer at -1°F or -20°C	60 days after preparation	Thaw at room temperature; Reheat in pot or microwave

Note: Vegan ranch, sour cream, and/or jalapeños are also great toppings!

Tip: Press the water out of the tofu before cooking. This will reduce the time it needs to brown.

13. Vegan Goulash

Nutrition Information
(per serving)

- Calories: 591 kcal.
- Carbs: 83.8g.
- Fat: 18.7g.
- Protein: 16.5g.
- Fiber: 14.2g.
- Sugar: 20.4g.

INGREDIENTS:

- 5 tbsp. olive oil
- 12 onions (medium, finely chopped)
- 1 head garlic (minced)
- 4 red bell peppers (cored, chopped)
- 10 tomatoes (small, cubed)
- 4 tbsp. paprika powder
- ½ cup dry red wine
- 3-6 cups vegetable broth (page 17)
- 10 potatoes (medium, skinned, cubed)
- 1 (7oz.) pack tempeh (substitute with textured soy protein)
- Salt and pepper to taste
- ¼ cup fresh parsley (chopped)

Total number of ingredients: 12

METHOD:

1. Heat the olive oil, in a large pot over medium heat.
2. Sauté the onions until brown.
3. Add the minced garlic and stir for 1 minute.
4. Continue to add the chopped bell peppers and cook the ingredients for another 3 minutes while stirring.
5. Blend in the tomatoes, paprika powder, salt, pepper and the dry red wine.
6. Stir thoroughly while letting the mixture cook for another 2 minutes.
7. Add the vegetable broth and the potato cubes to the pot and stir to combine all ingredients.
8. Put a lid on the pot and allow the goulash to cook for another 5 minutes.
9. Turn the heat down to low and continue to gently cook the goulash for 15 minutes. The goulash will thicken and the potatoes will get cooked properly.
10. Add the tempeh and taste to see if the goulash needs more salt and pepper.
11. Let the goulash cook for another 15 minutes.
12. Check if the potatoes have softened with a fork. Cook the mixture a few minutes more if the potatoes are hard to penetrate.
13. Once the potatoes are soft, add the parsley, stir and take the goulash off the heat.
14. Allow the goulash to cool down for about 10 minutes and serve or allow the goulash to cool down longer before storing.

STORAGE INFORMATION:

Storage	Temperature	Expiration date	Preparation
Airtight container M/L	Fridge at 38 – 40°F or 3°C	3-4 days after preparation	Reheat in microwave
Airtight container M/L	Freezer at -1°F or -20°C	60 days after preparation	Thaw at room temperature. Reheat in microwave

14. Golden Tofu Noodle Bowl

Nutrition Information
(per serving)
- Calories: 547 kcal.
- Carbs: 63.3g.
- Fat: 22.4.
- Protein: 23.3g.
- Fiber: 9.3g.
- Sugar: 12.7g.

INGREDIENTS:
- 1½ cups brown rice or rice noodles
- 1 cup firm tofu (cubed)
- 2 tbsp. coconut oil
- 1 radish (sliced)
- 1 carrot (large, peeled)
- ½ cucumber (sliced)
- 1 cup edamame (shelled)
- ¼ cup pickled red cabbage (optional)
- Roasted sesame seeds (optional)

Soy hoisin sauce:
- 3 tbsp. hoisin sauce
- 1 tsp. sriracha (or tabasco)
- ¼ cup soy sauce
- 1 lime (squeezed)

Total number of ingredients: 13

METHOD:
1. Cook the rice (or noodles) according to the recipe or package instructions.
2. Put in all sauce ingredients into a small bowl and stir well. Set the sauce aside.
3. Boil some water in a medium pot.
4. Steam the edamame in a sieve above the boiling water for about 5 minutes and shell them.
5. Take a large skillet, put it on medium heat and add the coconut oil.
6. Stir fry the tofu for about 5 minutes until brown before stirring in the hoisin sauce.
7. Serve the cooked rice or noodles with the tofu and sauce in a bowl.
8. Top the dish with the steamed edamame, carrot, cucumber and raw radish.
9. Add the optional roasted sesame seeds and pickled red cabbage.
10. Serve and enjoy or store the fresh and cooked ingredients in multiple-compartment containers!

STORAGE INFORMATION:

Storage	Temperature	Expiration date	Preparation
3-section airtight container M/L or/and Ziploc bags	Fridge at 38 – 40°F or 3°C	4-5 days after preparation	Reheat in pot or microwave
3-section airtight container M/L or/and Ziploc bags	Freezer at -1°F or -20°C	60 days after preparation	Thaw at room temperature. Reheat in pot or microwave

Note: store the rice, tofu and vegetables in 3-section containers or separate containers. Serve the meal with some extra (fresh or premade) soy hoisin sauce to add more flavor!

15. Tempeh Curry

Serves: 4 | Prep Time: ~ 20 min |

Nutrition Information
(per serving)

- Calories: 411 kcal.
- Carbs: 44.5g.
- Fat: 13.7g.
- Protein: 27.5g.
- Fiber: 8.4g.
- Sugar: 4.4g.

INGREDIENTS:

- 15 oz. tempeh
- 2 cups quinoa
- ½ cup red bell pepper (chopped)
- ½ cup purple cabbage (shredded)
- ½ cup sweet potato (finely chopped)
- 2 cups kale (chopped)
- 2 cups broccoli florets (chopped, fresh or frozen)

Tempeh seasoning:
- 3 tbsp. soy sauce
- 3 tbsp. sesame oil
- 3 tsp. rice vinegar
- 1 tsp. chili flakes (optional)

Cashew Curry Sauce:
- ½ cup cashew cheese spread (page 25)
- ¼ cup coconut cream
- ¼ cup coconut milk
- 2 tbsp. soy sauce
- 3 tsp. rice vinegar
- 2 tsp. red curry paste

Total number of ingredients: 17

METHOD:

1. Prepare the quinoa according to the "Quinoa" on page 13.
2. Use a sharp cutting knife to cut the tempeh into small, thin squares.
3. Transfer the tempeh squares to a medium sized bowl.
4. Marinate the squares with soy sauce, sesame oil and rice vinegar.
5. Carefully stir the tempeh and allow the squares to sit in the seasoning for 10 minutes.
6. Stir-fry the marinated tempeh in a large skillet with the chopped bell pepper, cabbage and sweet potato for about 5 minutes.
7. Take the skillet off the heat and set the stir-fried tempeh and veggies aside.
8. Fill a large pot with water and bring it to a boil.
9. Steam or cook the chopped broccoli florets in a sieve for about 3 minutes and set aside.
10. Reuse the large pot and add all the curry sauce ingredients.
11. Put the pot on low heat and gently whisk the ingredients until a smooth creamy sauce has formed.
12. Stir in the freshly chopped kale, cooked broccoli, fried tempeh and veggies.
13. Add the quinoa to the curry mixture in the pot and mix.
14. Enjoy warm or store for later!

STORAGE INFORMATION:

Storage	Temperature	Expiration date	Preparation
Airtight container M/L	Fridge at 38 – 40°F or 3°C	2-3 days after preparation	Reheat in microwave
Airtight container M/L	Freezer at -1°F or -20°C	60 days after preparation	Thaw at room temperature. Reheat in microwave

WHOLE FOOD DINNERS

1. Crunchy Sesame Tofu

Nutrition Information
(per serving)

- Calories: 654 kcal.
- Carbs 35.4g.
- Fat: 41.9.
- Protein: 33.9g.
- Fiber: 9.1g.
- Sugar: 22g.

INGREDIENTS:

- 3 tbsp. sesame oil
- 2 cups firm tofu (cubed)
- ¼ cup soy sauce
- 2 zucchinis (medium, sliced into noodles)
- 2 tbsp. roasted sesame seeds (optional)
- 1 green onion (sliced, optional)

Sesame peanut topping:

- ½ cup peanut butter
- ¼ cup soy sauce
- ¼ cup rice vinegar
- 2 tsp. chili flakes
- 2 tbsp. maple syrup
- 5g. of fresh ginger (peeled, chopped)
- 3 garlic cloves

Total number of ingredients: 13

METHOD:

1. Put a large skillet on medium heat and add 2 tablespoons of sesame oil.
2. Put in the cubed tofu and sauté these until light brown.
3. Add the first ¼ cup of soy sauce and stir well.
4. Turn the heat down to low and allow the tofu to absorb the soy sauce until the tofu is slightly crisp.
5. Put the crispy tofu aside for later.
6. Take a blender and mix all the sesame peanut topping ingredients.
7. Mix the tofu with the sesame peanut topping.
8. Serve the raw zucchini noodles with the crispy tofu and sauce in a medium bowl.
9. Top the dish with the optional roasted sesame seeds and green onion slices.
10. Serve and enjoy right away or store the ingredients separately!

STORAGE INFORMATION:

Storage	Temperature	Expiration date	Preparation
3-section airtight container M/L or/and Ziploc bags	Fridge at 38 – 40°F or 3°C	4-5 days after preparation	Reheat in pot or microwave
3-section airtight container M/L or/and Ziploc bags	Freezer at -1°F or -20°C	60 days after preparation	Thaw at room temperature. Reheat in pot or microwave

Note: keep the zucchini noodles, tofu and toppings in a 3 or 4-section container, separate containers and/ or Ziploc bags.

2. Bean Burritos

Nutrition Information
(per serving)
- Calories: 408 kcal.   - Protein: 14.5g.
- Carbs: 76.25g.   - Fiber: 14.4g.
- Fat: 11.4g.   - Sugar: 4.6g.

INGREDIENTS:

- ½ cup dry black beans
- 1 cup dry quinoa
- 4 tortillas (large, whole wheat)
- 2 tbsp. olive oil
- 3 cloves garlic (minced)
- 1 zucchini (medium, quartered vertically)
- 1 green bell pepper (medium, pitted, diced)
- 1 tomato (medium, diced)
- 1 (100g) can sweet corn (drained)
- 1 tbsp. fresh lime juice
- Salt and pepper to taste

Optional: special spiced pesto
- 1 cup cilantro leaves
- ¼ cup cashews (raw)
- ¼ cup olive oil
- 1 clove garlic
- 1 jalapeño pepper (small, seeded)
- 1 tbsp. lime juice
- Salt and pepper to taste

Total number of ingredients: 18

METHOD:

1. Prepare the black beans according to the "Soaking and cooking time per bean or legume" on page 7.
2. Cook the quinoa according to the "Quinoa" on page 13.
3. Put a large skillet on medium heat and add the olive oil.
4. Add the garlic, zucchini and bell pepper.
5. Stir the vegetables for about 10 minutes while adding the tomato and corn.
6. Transfer the vegetables to a large bowl.
7. Top the veggies with salt and black pepper to taste and stir well.
8. Prepare the optional pesto by blending all the special spiced pesto ingredients in a blender or food processor.
9. Top the veggies in the bowl with the optional pesto and stir well for about 2 minutes.
10. Scoop a portion of cooked beans and quinoa onto a tortilla.
11. Add some of the vegetable mixture with the optional pesto to the tortilla.
12. Top the mixture with some fresh lime juice.
13. Wrap the tortilla tightly and enjoy or store!

STORAGE INFORMATION:

Storage	Temperature	Expiration date	Preparation
Airtight container M/L or aluminum foil.	Fridge at 38 – 40°F or 3°C	3-4 days after preparation	Reheat in microwave
Airtight container M/L or aluminum foil.	Freezer at -1°F or -20°C	60 days after preparation	Thaw at room temperature. Reheat in microwave

Tip: wrap each prepared burrito in aluminum foil before storing in a storage container or Ziploc bag. WARNING: Do NOT microwave aluminum foil!

3. Cashew Spaghetti with Asparagus

Serves: 4 | Prep Time: ~20 min |

Nutrition Information
(per serving)
- Calories: 495 kcal.
- Carbs: 53.7g.
- Fat: 23.6g.
- Protein: 17g.
- Fiber: 11g.
- Sugar: 7g.

INGREDIENTS:

- 1 lb. whole-wheat spaghetti
- 5 tsp. olive oil
- 1 onion (large, chopped)
- 6 cloves garlic (chopped)
- 1 cup cashews (raw)
- 1 cup hot water
- 1 tbsp. tahini
- 1 lemon (medium, juiced)
- 1 tbsp. Dijon mustard
- 1 tbsp. nutritional yeast
- ½ tbsp. smoked paprika powder
- ½ tbsp. sweet paprika powder
- ¼ tsp. nutmeg
- 1 cup almond milk (unsweetened)
- 2 cups asparagus (chopped)
- ½ cup peas
- Salt and pepper to taste

Total number of ingredients: 17

METHOD:

1. Fill a large pot with water, add some salt and bring it to a boil.
2. Cook the whole-wheat spaghetti according to the instructions or for 10-14 minutes.
3. In the meantime, take a medium skillet and add 3 tablespoons olive oil.
4. Put the skillet on medium heat and fry the onions and garlic until softened.
5. Blend the raw cashews with hot water in a blender for about 5 minutes.
6. Add the sautéed garlic, onion, tahini, lemon juice, Dijon mustard, yeast, paprika powders, nutmeg, salt and pepper to the blender.
7. Blend all these ingredients until the mixture has the consistency of a sauce.
8. Transfer the sauce to the previously used skillet and put it on medium heat.
9. Add the almond milk to the sauce and stir until the creamy substance has the desired thickness.
10. Drain the pasta and set it aside.
11. Fill up the pot with fresh water and bring to a boil.
12. Cook the chopped asparagus and peas with the remaining 2 tablespoons olive oil.
13. Drain the water from the pot after the vegetables are cooked.
14. Add the cooked spaghetti back in and stir well.
15. Pour the creamy sauce on top when serving.
16. Mix well and add more spices, salt or pepper to taste.
17. Enjoy!

STORAGE INFORMATION:

Storage	Temperature	Expiration date	Preparation
Airtight container L	Fridge at 38 – 40°F or 3°C	4-5 days after preparation	Reheat in pot or microwave
Airtight container L	Freezer at -1°F or -20°C	60 days after preparation	Thaw at room temperature. Reheat in pot or microwave

4. 'Veggieful' Chili

Serves: 8 | Prep Time: ~15 min |

Nutrition Information
(per serving)
- Calories: 256 kcal.
- Carbs: 43.6g.
- Fat: 4.5gr.
- Protein: 13g.
- Fiber: 16.8g.
- Sugar: 8.5g.

INGREDIENTS:
- 1½ cups raw black beans
- 1½ cups raw kidney beans
- 2 tbsp. olive oil
- 2 red onions (medium, diced)
- 1 clove garlic (minced)
- 2 tsp. cumin
- ¼ tsp. cayenne pepper
- 2 tsp. oregano
- 1 zucchini (medium, diced)
- 1 yellow squash (small, diced)
- 1 red bell pepper (small, diced)
- 2 cups water
- 1 jalapeño (medium, diced)
- 1 cup tomato paste
- 1 (200g) can sweet corn (drained)
- 1 tbsp. chili powder
- Salt and pepper to taste

Total number of ingredients: 17

METHOD:
1. Prepare the black and kidney beans according to the"Soaking and cooking time per bean or legume" on page 7.
2. Take a large pan, put it on medium high heat and add the olive oil.
3. Sautee the diced red onions for about 5 minutes.
4. Blend in the garlic, cumin, cayenne pepper, oregano while stirring.
5. Add the diced zucchini, squash, bell pepper and stir again.
6. Allow the mixture to fry for a few minutes while constantly stirring.
7. Lower the heat to medium and add 2 cups of water, jalapeño, tomato paste, corn and cooked beans.
8. Stir well while adding the chili powder, salt and optionally more pepper to taste.
9. Reduce the heat to low, cover the pan and let the chili simmer for about 20 minutes.
10. Add more spices like cumin, oregano, chili powder or cayenne pepper to taste.
11. Serve and enjoy warm or allow the chili to cool down to store it in containers!

STORAGE INFORMATION:

Storage	Temperature	Expiration date	Preparation
2-compartment airtight container M	Fridge at 38 – 40°F or 3°C	3-4 days after preparation	Reheat in microwave
2-compartment airtight container M	Freezer at -1°F or -20°C	60 days after preparation	Thaw at room temperature. Reheat in microwave

Note: keep the black beans separated from the chili. Use a 2-compartment or two separate containers to store each meal.

5. Spicy Beet Bowl

Serves: 3 | Prep Time: ~15 min |

Nutrition Information
(per serving)

- Calories: 445 kcal.
- Carbs: 48.7g.
- Fat: 20.5g.
- Protein: 16.4g.
- Fiber: 17.3g.
- Sugar: 14.2g.

INGREDIENTS:
Bowl contents:

- 1 cup dry sushi rice
- 3 Chioggia beets (medium, sliced)
- ¼ lemon (fresh, juice)
- 2-4 tsp. olive oil
- 2g. fresh ginger (peeled, cut)
- 2 cups edamame beans
- 2 tsp. olive oil
- 2 green onions (sliced)
- 1 carrot (big, sliced)
- Salt to taste
- 3 tsp. roasted sesame seeds (optional)
- Handful nori flakes (optional)

Wasabi avocado paste:

- 1 avocado (big, peeled and pitted)
- ¼ lemon (fresh, juice)
- 2 tsp. wasabi powder
- Salt to taste

Total number of ingredients: 16

METHOD:

1. Preheat oven to 375°F or 190°C.
2. Cook the sushi rice according to the "Method for long-grain rice:" on page 11.
3. Wrap the sliced Chioggia beets in aluminum foil.
4. Transfer the packed beet slices to a baking tray and put it in the oven.
5. Roast the beets for about 45 minutes. Take the tray out and set it aside.
6. Scoop out the avocado flesh and cut it into small pieces.
7. Transfer the avocado to a small bowl and add half of the lemon juice, wasabi powder and salt to taste.
8. Mash until the avocado mixture is creamy and set aside.
9. Take a large bowl and mix in the other half of the lemon juice, olive oil, ginger and more salt to taste.
10. Take the foil off the roasted beets and put the slices in this large bowl.
11. Boil some water in a medium pot.
12. Steam the edamame beans topped with a pinch of salt in a sieve above the boiling water for about 5 minutes.
13. Top the edamame with a pinch of olive oil and salt to taste. Set the beans aside.
14. Take a medium bowl for serving and add the rice, beets and steamed edamame.
15. Top the dish with the wasabi avocado paste, green onion slices, carrot slices, optional roasted sesame seeds and nori flakes.
16. Serve and enjoy or store the ingredients separately for another day!

STORAGE INFORMATION:

Storage	Temperature	Expiration date	Preparation
4-section airtight container and/ or Ziploc bags	Fridge at 38 – 40°F or 3°C	2 days after preparation	Reheat in pot or microwave and add toppings after heating.
4-section airtight container and/ or Ziploc bags	Freezer at -1°F or -20°C	60 days after preparation	Thaw at room temperature. Reheat in pot or microwave and add toppings after heating.

Note: keep the rice, roasted beet slices, vegetables and the avocado wasabi paste in a 4-section container, separate containers and/or Ziploc bags.

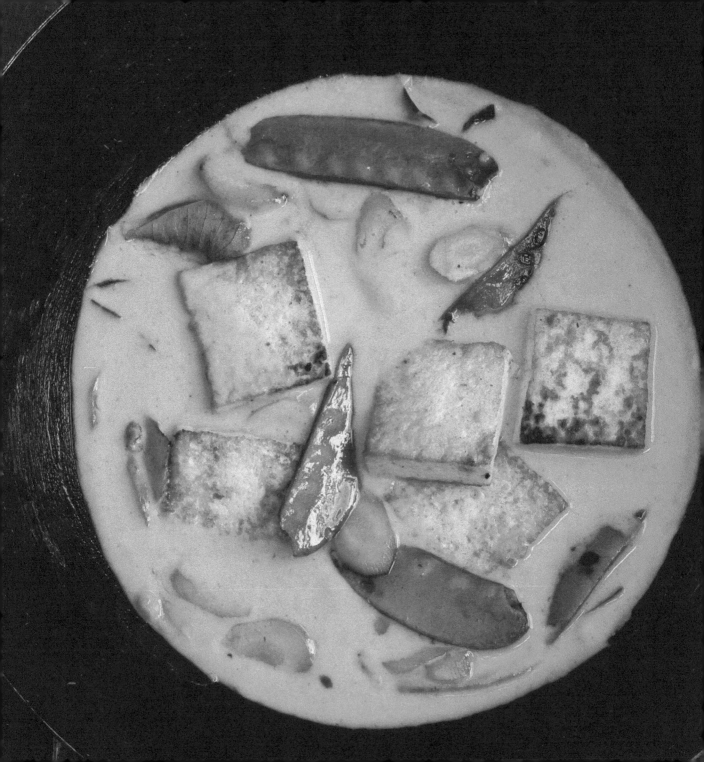

6. Coconut Tofu Curry

Serves: 2 | Prep Time: ~30 min |

Nutrition Information
(per serving)

- Calories: 449 kcal
- Carbs: 38.7 g.
- Fat: 23 g.
- Protein: 21.8 g.
- Fiber: 8.6 g.
- Sugar: 18.8 g.

INGREDIENTS:

- 1 14-oz. block firm tofu
- 2 tsp. coconut oil
- 1 medium sweet onion (diced)
- 1 13-oz. can reduced-fat coconut milk
- 1 cup tomatoes (fresh, diced)
- 1 cup snap peas
- 1½ inch ginger (finely minced)
- 1 tsp. curry powder
- 1 tsp. tumeric
- 1 tsp. cumin
- ½ tsp. red pepper flakes
- 1 tsp. agave nectar (or sweet substitute)
- Salt and pepper to taste

Total number of ingredients: 14

METHOD:

1. Cut the tofu into ½-inch cubes.
2. Heat the coconut oil in a large skillet over medium-high heat.
3. Add the tofu and cook for about 5 minutes.
4. Stir in the garlic and diced onions, and sauté until the onions are transparent (for about 5 to 10 minutes); add the ginger while stirring.
5. Add in the coconut milk, tomatoes, agave nectar, snap peas, and remaining spices.
6. Combine thoroughly, cover, and cook on low heat; remove after 10 minutes of cooking.
7. For serving, scoop the curry into a bowl or over rice.
8. Enjoy right away, or, store the curry in an airtight container to enjoy later!

STORAGE INFORMATION:

Storage	Temperature	Expiration date	Preparation
Airtight container M/L	Fridge at 38 – 40°F or 3°C	4-5 days after preparation	Reheat in pot or microwave
Airtight container M/L	Freezer at -1°F or -20°C	60 days after preparation	Thaw at room temperature; Reheat in pot or microwave

Note: Add any other fresh vegetables you have on hand to this dish!

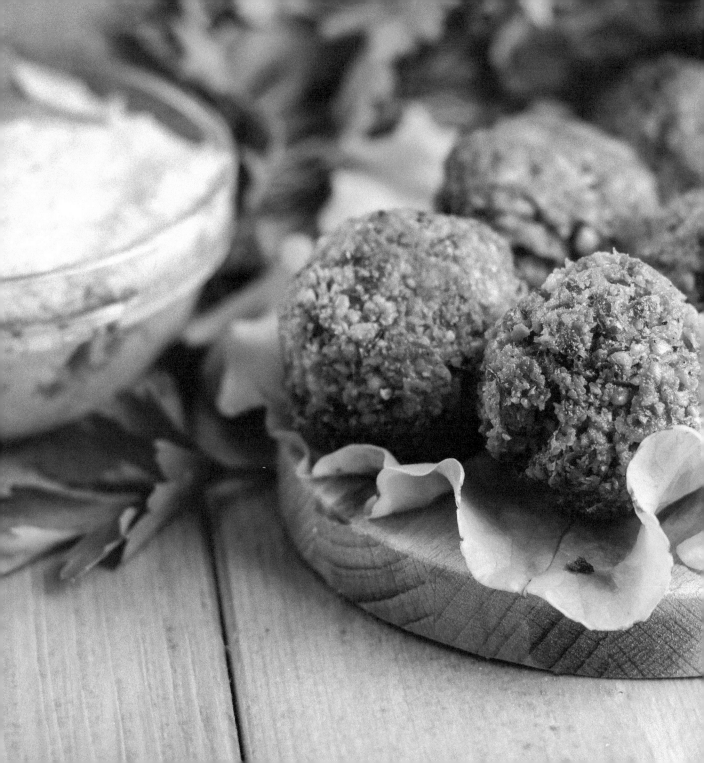

7. Tahini Falafels

Serves: 4 | Prep Time: ~30 min |

Nutrition Information
(per serving)
- Calories: 220 kcal
- Carbs: 28 g.
- Fat: 7.3 g.
- Protein: 10.5 g.
- Fiber: 8 g.
- Sugar: 3.9 g.

INGREDIENTS:

- 2 cups dry chickpeas
- ½ cup dry black beans
- 2 cups broccoli florrets
- 1 garlic clove (minced)
- 2 tsp. cumin
- 1 tsp. olive oil
- ½ tsp. lemon juice
- ½ tsp. paprika
- ¼ tsp. tumeric
- Dash of salt
- 2 tbsp. tahini

Total number of ingredients: 11

METHOD:

1. Prepare the chickpeas according to the "Soaking and sprouting chia, hemp and flaxseeds" on page 10.
2. Prepare the black beans according to the "Soaking and cooking time per bean or legume" on page 7.
3. Preheat the oven to 400°F / 200°C.
4. Meanwhile, place the broccoli florrets in a large skillet and drizzle them with the olive oil and salt.
5. Roast the broccoli until the florets tender and brown, over medium-high heat, for 5 to 10 minutes; set aside and allow to cool a little.
6. Place the cooled broccoli with all the remaining ingredients—except the tahini—into a food processor. Blend on low for 2-3 minutes, until most large lumps are gone.
7. Line a baking pan with parchment paper. Press the falafel dough into 8 equal-sized patties, and place them evenly-spaced apart on the parchment.
8. Bake the falafels until they are brown and crisp on the outside, for roughly 10 to 15 minutes. Make sure to flip them halfway through to ensure even cooking.
9. Serve with tahini as topping, or, let the falafel cool down and store for later.

STORAGE INFORMATION:

Storage	Temperature	Expiration date	Preparation
Airtight container M/L	Fridge at 38 – 40°F or 3°C	3-4 days after preparation	Reheat in pot or microwave
Airtight container M/L	Freezer at -1°F or -20°C	60 days after preparation	Thaw at room temperature; Reheat in pot or microwave

Note: These falafels also taste great in gluten-free pitas and topped with vegan garlic sauce!

Tip: The falafel will taste dry if the mixture is too chunky, and it will fall apart if blended for too long. Aim for a mixture that has some mid-sized lumps remaining.

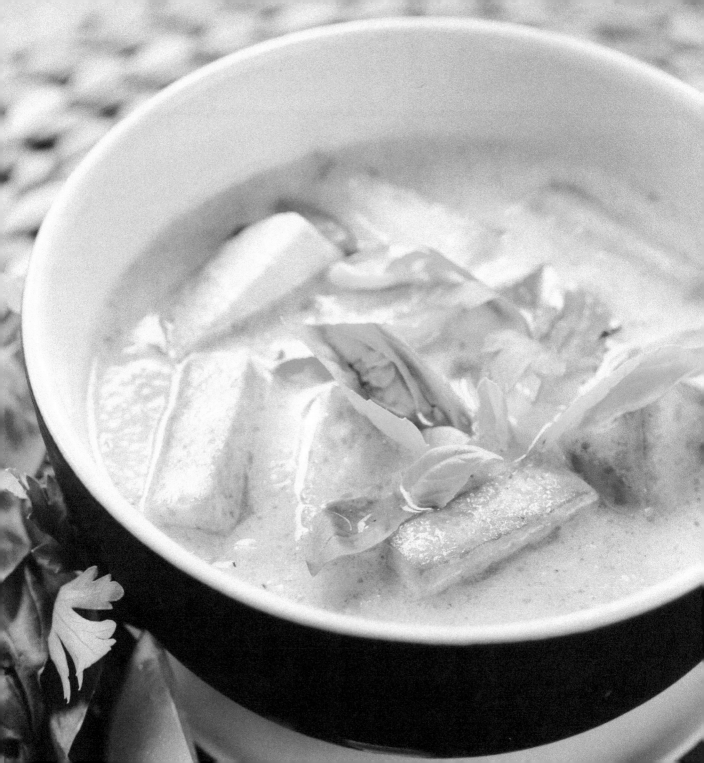

8. Green Thai Curry

Nutrition Information
(per serving)

- Calories: 327 kcal
- Carbs: 35.6 g.
- Fat: 14.9 g.
- Protein: 12.5 g.
- Fiber: 6.8 g.
- Sugar: 10.5 g.

INGREDIENTS:

- 1 cup white rice
- ½ cup dry chickpeas
- 2 tbsp. olive oil
- 1 14-oz. package firm tofu (drained)
- 1 medium green bell pepper
- ½ white onion (diced)
- 2 tbsp. green curry paste
- 1 cup reduced-fat coconut milk
- 1 cup water (alternatively use vegetable broth (page 17))
- 1 cup peas (fresh or frozen)
- 1/3 cup fresh Thai basil (chopped)
- 2 tbsp. maple syrup (or other sweetener)
- ½ tsp. lime juice
- Dash of salt

Total number of ingredients: 14

METHOD:

1. Prepare the rice according to the "Method for long-grain rice:" on page 11.
2. Prepare the chickpeas according to "Soaking and sprouting chia, hemp and flaxseeds" on page 10.
3. Cut the tofu into ½-inch pieces.
4. Heat up the olive oil in a large skillet over medium-high heat and and fry the tofu about 3 minutes per side.
5. Remove the skillet from the stove and and set the tofu aside in a medium-sized bowl with the cooked chickpeas.
6. Using the same skillet over medium-high heat, add the bell pepper and onions and sauté until they are softened, for about 5 minutes.
7. Remove the skillet from the heat, add the green curry paste, vegetable broth, and coconut milk to the skillet.
8. Stir until the curry paste is well incorporated; then add the tofu, chickpeas, and peas to the mixture and cook for 10 more minutes.
9. Drop in the Thai basil, maple syrup, and salt, and bring the mixture back up to a low cooking bubble, stirring constantly for about 3 minutes. Remove from heat.
10. Serve with rice, topped with additional chopped Thai basil, or store for later!

STORAGE INFORMATION:

Storage	Temperature	Expiration date	Preparation
2-compartment Airtight container M/L	Fridge at 38 – 40°F or 3°C	3-4 days after preparation	Reheat in pot or microwave
2-compartment Airtight container M/L	Freezer at -1°F or -20°C	60 days after preparation	Thaw at room temperature; Reheat in pot or microwave

Note: Easily customize this dish by adding more vegetables you have on hand!

Tip: Small cubes of tofu will cook too quickly for this dish. Make sure they're at least half an inch for the best results. Store the curry and rice separately.

9. Cuban Tempeh Buddha Bowl

Nutrition Information
(per serving)
- Calories: 343 kcal
- Carbs: 27.4 g.
- Fat: 18.3 g.
- Protein: 17.1 g.
- Fiber: 4.7 g.
- Sugar: 0.7 g.

INGREDIENTS:
- 1 cup basmati rice
- 1 cup dry black beans
- 1 14-oz. package tempeh (thinly sliced)
- 1 cup water, alternatively use vegetable broth (page 17))
- 2 tsp. chili powder
- 1 tsp. lime juice
- 1¼ tsp. cumin
- 1 pinch of salt
- 1 tsp. tumeric
- 2 tbsp. coconut oil
- 1 medium avocado (pitted, peeled, diced)

Total number of ingredients: 11

METHOD:
1. Prepare the rice according the "Method for short-grain rice:" on page 12.
2. Prepare the black beans according the "Soaking and cooking time per bean or legume" on page 7.
3. Mix the vegetable broth, chili powder, cumin, turmeric, salt, and lime juice in a large bowl.
4. Add the tempeh and let it marinate in the fridge for up to 3 hours.
5. Heat up a frying pan with the coconut oil on medium-high heat and add the tempeh with the marinating juices.
6. Bring everything to a boil, turn down the heat, and cook over low heat until the broth is gone—10 to 15 minutes.
7. Serve the tempeh in a bowl with a scoop of rice, and top with the cooked black beans and diced avocado.

STORAGE INFORMATION:

Storage	Temperature	Expiration date	Preparation
Airtight container M/L	Fridge at 38 – 40°F or 3°C	3-4 days after preparation	Reheat in pot or microwave
Airtight container M/L	Freezer at -1°F or -20°C	60 days after preparation	Thaw at room temperature; Reheat in pot or microwave

Note: You can also top these buddha bowls with some cherry tomatoes, salsa, and/ or vegan sour cream.

Tip: Undercooked tempeh will be chewy; cook the slices until they are brown and crispy for the best flavor.

10. Baked Enchilada Bowls

Serves: 4 | Prep Time: ~60 min |

Nutrition Information
(per serving)
- Calories: 417 kcal
- Carbs: 34.6 g.
- Fat: 27.1 g.
- Protein: 15.6 g.
- Fiber: 7.2 g.
- Sugar: 6.9 g.

INGREDIENTS:
- 1 cup dry black beans
- 1 large sweet potato
- 4 tbsp. olive oil
- 2 cups enchilada sauce (page 26)
- 1 green bell pepper (fresh or a frozen red/green mix)
- ½ purple onion (diced)
- 1 14-oz. package firm tofu
- ½ cup cashews (chopped)
- 1 tsp. cumin
- 1 tsp. paprika
- 1 tsp. garlic powder
- 1 tsp. salt
- ½ cup vegan cheese (page 25)
- 1 tbsp. chopped jalapeños (optional)

Total number of ingredients: 14

METHOD:
1. Prepare the black beans according to the "Soaking and cooking time per bean or legume" on page 7.
2. Preheat oven to 400°F / 200°C .
3. Cut the sweet potatoes into ¼-inch cubes and place them in a bowl with 2 tablespoons of the olive oil, the garlic powder and ½ teaspoon of salt; toss well and make sure the sweet potatoes get coated evenly.
4. Arrange the sweet potatoes in a single layer on a baking pan. Place the pan in the oven and bake until the potato cubes begin to soften, for 15-20 minutes.
5. Meanwhile, dice up the bell pepper, onion, and tofu into ¼-inch cubes and place all in the previously used bowl with the remaining olive oil, cashews and ½ teaspoon of salt.
6. Stir the ingredients thoroughly to make sure everything gets coated evenly.
7. After removing the potatoes from the oven, add the tofu, peppers, and onions to the baking pan and stir until combined.
8. Put the baking pan back into the oven for an additional 10 minutes, until the onions are browned and peppers are soft.
9. Remove the pan from the oven and place the contents into a casserole dish.
10. Add the cooked black beans, enchilada sauce, and spices to the casserole dish, mixing everything until it's evenly distributed.
11. Top with a layer of vegan cheese and return to oven until it is melted, around 15 minutes.
12. Serve in a bowl topped with the optional jalapeños, or store for later!

STORAGE INFORMATION:

Storage	Temperature	Expiration date	Preparation
Airtight container M/L	Fridge at 38 – 40°F or 3°C	4-5 days after preparation	Reheat in pot or microwave
Airtight container M/L	Freezer at -1°F or -20°C	60 days after preparation	Thaw at room temperature; Reheat in pot or microwave

Note: Raw purple onions, avocado slices, and/or salsa make great toppings.

Tip: Don't overcook the sweet potatoes! They'll continue cooking later in the recipe.

SNACKS FOR ENERGY AND RECOVERY

1. Gluten-Free Energy Crackers

Serves: 6 | Prep Time: ~60 min |

Nutrition Information
(per serving)

- Calories: 209 kcal
- Carbs: 10.3 g.
- Fat: 15.6 g.
- Protein: 6.9 g.
- Fiber: 6.3 g.
- Sugar: 0.7 g.

INGREDIENTS:

- ¼ cup flax seeds
- ¼ cup chia seeds
- ¾ cup water
- 1 tbsp. garlic (minced)
- ½ tbsp. onion flakes (alternatively use onion powder)
- ½ cup pumpkin seeds (chopped)
- ¼ cup peanuts (crushed)
- ¼ cup cashews (crushed)
- ¼ cup sesame seeds
- ¼ tsp. paprika powder
- Salt and pepper to taste

Total number of ingredients: 12

METHOD:

1. Preheat the oven to 350°F / 175°C.
2. Take a large bowl and combine the water, garlic, onion flakes, and paprika. Whisk until everything is combined thoroughly.
3. Add the flax seeds, chia seeds, pumpkin seeds, peanuts, cashews, and sesame seeds to the bowl.
4. Stir everything well, while adding pinches of salt and pepper to taste, until it is thoroughly combined.
5. Line a baking sheet with parchment paper and spread out the mixture in a thin and even layer across the parchment paper.
6. Bake for 20-25 minutes.
7. Remove the pan from the oven and flip over the flat chunk so that the other side can crisp.
8. Cut the chunk into squares or triangles, depending on preference and put the pan back into the oven and bake until the bars have turned golden brown, around 30 minutes.
9. Allow the crackers to cool before serving or storing. Enjoy!

STORAGE INFORMATION:

Storage	Temperature	Expiration date	Preparation
Airtight container L	Fridge at 38 – 40°F or 3°C	4-5 days after preparation	Reheat in pot or microwave
Airtight container L	Freezer at -1°F or -20°C	60 days after preparation	Thaw at room temperature

Note: Experiment with extra seeds, nuts, and spices. Try different combinations for an endless variety of energy cracker flavors!

Tip: A thin layer of the mixture will make thin crackers, while a thicker layer will make thicker crackers. Thicker crackers will take longer to crisp in the oven.

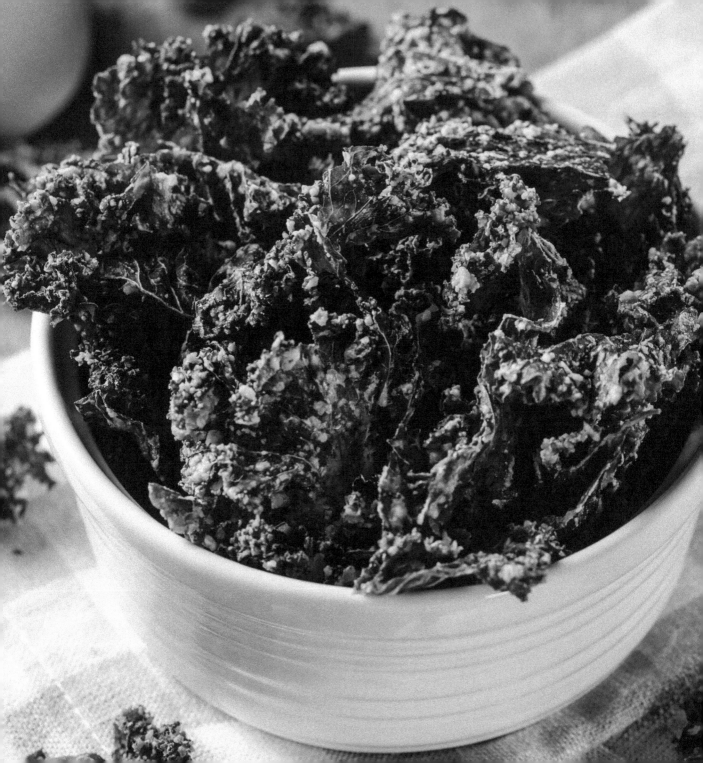

2. Mexikale Crisps

Serves: 2 | Prep Time: ~10 min |

Nutrition Information
(per serving)
- Calories: 313 kcal.
- Carbs: 33.4g.
- Fat: 14.6g.
- Protein: 12g.
- Fiber: 7g.
- Sugar: 0.3g.

INGREDIENTS:

- 8 cups kale leaves (large, chopped)
- 2 tbsp. avocado oil
- 2 tbsp. nutritional yeast
- 1 tsp. garlic powder
- 1 tsp. ground cumin
- ½ tsp. chili powder
- 1 tsp. dried oregano
- 1 tsp. dried cilantro
- Salt and pepper to taste

Total number of ingredients: 9

METHOD:

1. Preheat the oven to 350°F or 175°C.
2. Line a baking tray with parchment paper and set it aside.
3. Absorb any remaining water from the chopped kale leaves with paper towels.
4. Place the chopped leaves in a large bowl and add the avocado oil, yeast and seasonings.
5. Mix and shake well before adding more yeast and extra seasonings if desired. Mix all the ingredients again.
6. Spread out the kale chips on the baking tray.
7. Bake the kale in the oven for 10-15 minutes. Check every minute after the 10-minute mark until the preferred crispiness is reached.
8. Take the tray out of the oven and set it aside to cool down.
9. Serve and enjoy or store in a container for later!

STORAGE INFORMATION:

Storage	Temperature	Expiration date	Preparation
Airtight container M	Fridge at 38 – 40°F or 3°C	4-5 days after preparation	
Airtight container M	Freezer at -1°F or -20°C	60 days after preparation	Thaw at room temperature.

3. Flaxseed Yogurt

Serves: 4| Prep Time: ~5 min |

Nutrition Information
(per serving)
- Calories: 220 kcal.
- Carbs: 9.2g
- Fat: 16.9g
- Protein: 10g
- Fiber: 7.4g
- Sugar: 0.7g

INGREDIENTS:
- 2 cups water
- ½ cup hemp seeds
- ½ cup flax seeds
- 1 cup almond milk
- 2 tsp. psyllium husk
- ¼ cup lemon juice
- ¼ tsp. stevia

Total number of ingredients: 7

METHOD:
1. Soak the flax seeds according the "Soaking" on page 6. Drain the excess water.
2. Add 1 cup of boiling water to a heat resistant blender.
3. Continue to add the dry and soaked seeds.
4. Blend the ingredients for about 4 minutes.
5. Pour another cup of water, the almond milk and psyllium husk in the blender. Blend the mix again for 30 seconds.
6. Finally, add the lemon juice and stevia. Blend for another few seconds.
7. Pour the flaxseed yogurt into a container and put it in the fridge.
8. Serve the flaxseed yogurt chilled and enjoy or divide the yogurt for storing.

STORAGE INFORMATION:

Storage	Temperature	Expiration date	Preparation
Airtight container M	Fridge at 38 – 40°F or 3°C	3-4 days after preparation	
Airtight container M	Freezer at -1°F or -20°C	60 days after preparation	Thaw in fridge.

Tip: the ingredients listed are good to produce 4 portions. Divide the yogurt over 4 airtight containers to serve or store the yogurt in portion sizes.

4. Overnight Cookie Dough Oats

Nutrition Information
(per serving)
- Calories: 316 kcal
- Carbs: 22.7 g.
- Fat: 11.3 g.
- Protein: 30.7 g.
- Fiber: 4.2 g.
- Sugar: 1.3 g.

INGREDIENTS:

- 1 cup almond milk (sweetened)
- ½ cup quick or rolled oats
- 2 scoops vegan protein powder (vanilla flavor)
- 1 tbsp. flaxseeds
- 1 tbsp. peanut butter (page 24)
- 1 tbsp. maple syrup (optional)
- 1 tbsp. carob chips (optional)

Total number of ingredients: 7

METHOD:

1. Take a lidded bowl or jar and add the oats, flaxseed, protein powder, and almond milk.
2. Stir until everything is thoroughly combined and the mixture looks runny; if not, add a little more almond milk.
3. Blend in the peanut butter with a spoon until everything is mixed well.
4. Place or close the lid on the bowl or jar and transfer it to the refrigerator.
5. Allow the jar to sit overnight—or for at least five hours—so the flavors can set.
6. Serve the dough oats, and if desired, topped with the optional carob chips and a small cap of maple syrup.
7. Enjoy immediately, or store without the optional ingredients in an airtight container.

STORAGE INFORMATION:

Storage	Temperature	Expiration date	Preparation
Airtight container M/L	Fridge at 38 – 40°F or 3°C	3-4 days after preparation	Consume chilled
Airtight container M/L	Freezer at -1°F or -20°C	60 days after preparation	Thaw at room temperature

Note: Make sure the oats are certified gluten-free for a gluten-free snack!

Tip: You can substitute the peanut butter with almond or cashew butter. Replacing the butter will also result in a creamy thick mixture.

5. Hazelnut & Chocolate Bars

Serves: 4 | Prep Time: ~15 min |

Nutrition Information
(per serving)
- Calories: 296 kcal
- Carbs: 21.3 g.
- Fat: 14.2 g.
- Protein: 20.6 g.
- Fiber: 3 g.
- Sugar: 12.7 g.

INGREDIENTS:
- 1 cup vegan chocolate protein powder
- ¼ cup hazelnuts (chopped)
- ¼ cup unsweetened cocoa powder
- 1/3 cup almond milk
- ¼ cup cashew butter
- 3 tbsp. brown rice syrup

Total number of ingredients: 6

METHOD:
1. In a large bowl, add the protein powder, cocoa, and hazelnuts; mix with a whisk to combine evenly.
2. Continue by adding the almond milk, cashew butter, and brown rice syrup; use the whisk or a small spatula to combine all ingredients thoroughly. Eventually the mixture should feel doughy and slightly sticky to the touch.
3. Lay out a sheet of parchment paper on a baking tray and place the dough in the middle. Press it out with your hands or a rolling pin until it's a ½-inch-thick square.
4. Put the baking tray in the fridge for 4 hours, or the freezer for 1½ hours.
5. Slice the chunk into 8 equal bars, and then serve and enjoy. Or, store for another day!

STORAGE INFORMATION:

Storage	Temperature	Expiration date	Preparation
Airtight container M/L or Ziploc bag	Fridge at 38 – 40°F or 3°C	4-5 days after preparation	
Airtight container M/L or Ziploc bag	Freezer at -1°F or -20°C	60 days after preparation	Thaw at room temperature

Note: Garnish with crushed hazelnuts or almonds for more crunch!

Tip: If the dough is too wet or sticky, add more cocoa or protein powder until you can handle it easily.

6. Chewy Almond Butter Balls

Serves: 2 | Prep Time: ~15 min |

Nutrition Information
(per serving)
- Calories: 329 kcal
- Carbs: 24.6 g.
- Fat: 16.5 g.
- Protein: 20.6 g.
- Fiber: 1 g.
- Sugar: 15.2 g.

INGREDIENTS:

- 2 tbsp. maple syrup
- ½ cup vegan protein powder (vanilla or chocolate flavor)
- ¼ cup almond butter
- 1 tbsp. pure vanilla extract
- 1 cup puffy rice cereal
- 1 tbsp. carob chips

Total number of ingredients: 6

METHOD:

1. Take a large bowl and thoroughly mix the maple syrup, protein powder, almond butter, and vanilla.
2. Microwave the bowl until the ingredients are heated through and the syrup and butter are melted, for about 40 seconds.
3. Add the puffy rice cereal and carob chips. Stir everything together evenly one more time.
4. Line a sheet pan with parchment paper, and using a spoon, scoop out the mixture and shape it into small-to-medium sized balls with your hands.
5. Press these balls firmly together to prevent crumbling and place them onto the pan with parchment paper.
6. Put the pan in the freezer for about 1 hour, or leave in the fridge for 4 hours.
7. Enjoy the balls cold or thawed at room temperature. Alternatively, store them in a container or Ziploc bag to enjoy later.

STORAGE INFORMATION:

Storage	Temperature	Expiration date	Preparation
Airtight container M/L or Ziploc bag	Fridge at 38 – 40°F or 3°C	3-4 days after preparation	Enjoy chilled or at room temperature
Airtight container M/L or Ziploc bag	Freezer at -1°F or -20°C	60 days after preparation	Thaw in the fridge or at room temperature

Note: Substitute a gluten-free version of the puffy rice cereal in this easy snack.

Tip: Almond or peanut butter will hold these treats together better than creamier butters like cashew.

7. Cranberry Vanilla Protein Bars

Serves: 4 | Prep Time: ~15 min |

Nutrition Information
(per serving)
- Calories: 243 kcal
- Carbs: 22.9 g.
- Fat: 9.6 g.
- Protein: 16.1 g.
- Fiber: 3.1 g.
- Sugar: 9.9 g.

INGREDIENTS:
- 1 cup old-fashioned oats
- 2 cups vegan protein powder
  (vanilla flavor)
- 1/3 cup shredded coconut
- ½ cup cashew butter
- ½ cup dried cranberries
- ¼ cup maple syrup
- ¼ cup chia seeds
- 1 tbsp. almond or soy milk
- 1 tbsp. pure vanilla extract

Total number of ingredients: 9

METHOD:
1. Line a square 8x8" baking dish with parchment paper and set it aside.
2. Add the oats, protein powder, and shredded coconut to a food processor and blend until they resemble a fine powder.
3. Transfer the blended ingredients to a large mixing bowl and add the remaining ingredients; mix with a spoon until everything is thoroughly combined.
4. Move the dough to the baking dish and press it down evenly until flattened as much as possible.
5. Place the dish into the freezer until set and firm, around 1½ hours.
6. To serve, slice the chunk into 8 even bars, and enjoy, share, or store!

STORAGE INFORMATION:

Storage	Temperature	Expiration date	Preparation
Airtight container M/L or Ziploc bag	Fridge at 38 – 40°F or 3°C	6-7 days after preparation	Serve chilled or at room temperature
Airtight container M/L or Ziploc bag	Freezer at -1°F or -20°C	60 days after preparation	Thaw at room temperature

Note: Dried cherries also make a great addition to these bars!

Tip: Use another flavor plant-based protein powder to alter the taste of these bars.

8. Mocha Chocolate Brownie Bars

Serves: 3 | Prep Time: ~15 min |

Nutrition Information
(per serving)
- Calories: 213 kcal
- Carbs: 17.3 g.
- Fat: 3.8 g.
- Protein: 27.3 g.
- Fiber: 3.7 g.
- Sugar: 6.1 g.

INGREDIENTS:

- 2½ cups vegan protein powder
  (chocolate or vanilla)
- ½ cup cocoa powder
- ½ cup old-fashioned or quick oats
- 1 tsp. pure vanilla extract
- ¼ tsp. nutmeg
- 2 tbsp. agave nectar
- 1 cup brewed coffee (cold)

Total number of ingredients: 7

METHOD:

1. Line a square baking dish with parchment paper and set it aside.
2. Mix the dry ingredients together in a large bowl.
3. Slowly incorporate the agave nectar, vanilla extract, and cold coffee while stirring constantly until all the lumps in the mixture have disappeared.
4. Pour the batter into the dish, while making sure to press it into the corners.
5. Place the dish into the refrigerator until firm, or for about 4 hours. Alternatively use the freezer for just 1 hour.
6. Slice the chunk into 6 even squares, and enjoy, share, or store!

STORAGE INFORMATION:

Storage	Temperature	Expiration date	Preparation
Airtight container M/L or Ziploc bag	Fridge at 38 – 40°F or 3°C	4-5 days after preparation	Serve chilled
Airtight container M/L or Ziploc bag	Freezer at -1°F or -20°C	60 days after preparation	Thaw at room temperature

Note: These brownies are even better when they're garnished with crushed hazelnuts or almonds!

Tip: Press the batter down firmly in the dish with a spoon to remove any air bubbles.

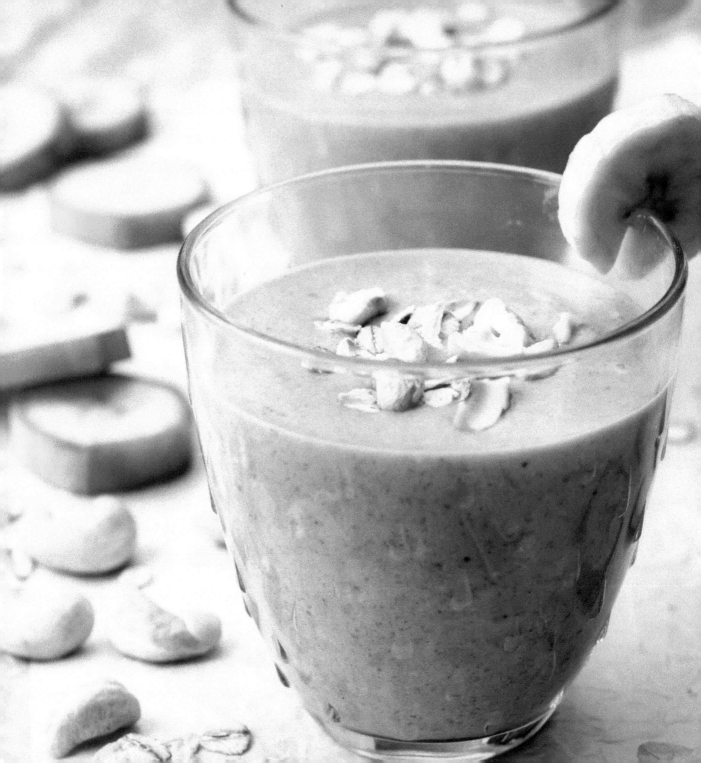

9. High Protein Cake Batter Smoothie

Serves: 2 | Prep Time: ~10 min |

Nutrition Information
(per serving)
- Calories: 241 kcal
- Carbs: 27.2 g.
- Fat: 7.6 g.
- Protein: 16 g.
- Fiber: 2.5 g.
- Sugar: 12.4 g.

INGREDIENTS:

- 1 large banana (frozen)
- 1 cup almond milk (alternatively use soy milk)
- ¼ cup quick oats
- 4 tbsp. vegan protein powder (chocolate flavor)
- 1 tbsp. cashew butter
- 1 tsp. cinnamon
- 1 tsp. pure vanilla extract
- ¼ tsp. nutmeg

Total number of ingredients: 8

METHOD:
1. Mix the oats and almond milk in a small bowl or jar.
2. Place the bowl in the fridge until the oats have softened, for about 1 hour.
3. Add the oats and milk mixture along with the remaining ingredients to a blender.
4. Blend on high speed until it is smooth and all lumps have disappeared.
5. Serve in tall glasses with an extra sprinkle of cinnamon on top, or store to enjoy later.

STORAGE INFORMATION:

Storage	Temperature	Expiration date	Preparation
Airtight thermos, cup, or jar	Fridge at 38 – 40°F or 3°C	2-3 days after preparation	Serve chilled
Airtight container S/M or jar	Freezer at -1°F or -20°C	60 days after preparation	Thaw in the fridge

Note: Other butters, like almond or peanut butter, will also work in this smoothie.

Tip: Soaking the oats prevents them from becoming gritty after blending.

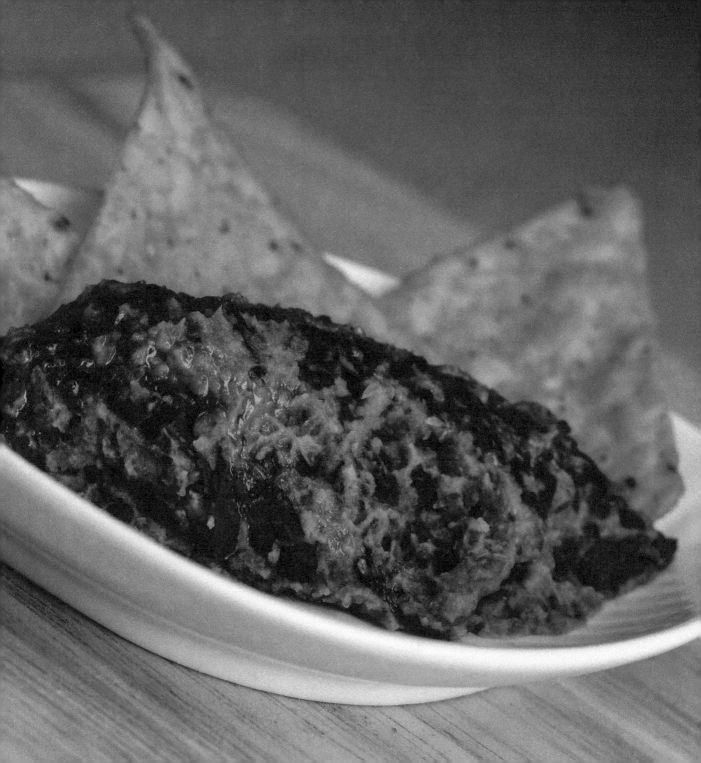

10. High Protein Black Bean Dip

Serves: 3 | Prep Time: ~10 min |

Nutrition Information
(per serving)

- Calories: 398 kcal
- Carbs: 63 g.
- Fat: 6.6 g.
- Protein: 21.3 g.
- Fiber: 16 g.
- Sugar: 3.5 g.

INGREDIENTS:

- 4 cups black beans (cooked, rinsed, drained)
- 2 tbsp. minced garlic
- 2 tbsp. Italian seasoning
- 2 tbsp. onion powder
- 1 tbsp. olive oil
- 1 tbsp. lemon juice
- ¼ tsp. salt + salt to taste

Total number of ingredients: 7

METHOD:

1. Place black beans in a large bowl and mash them with a fork until everything is mostly smooth.
2. Stir in the remaining ingredients and incorporate thoroughly. The mixture should be smooth and creamy.
3. Add some additional salt and lemon juice to taste and serve at room temperature.

STORAGE INFORMATION:

Storage	Temperature	Expiration date	Preparation
Airtight container S/M/L	Fridge at 38 – 40°F or 3°C	5 days after preparation	Reheat in microwave or serve cold
Airtight container S/M/L	Freezer at -1°F or -20°C	30 days after preparation	Reheat in microwave or serve cold

Note: Serve with slices of broccoli, carrots, and celery for a classic veggie dip.

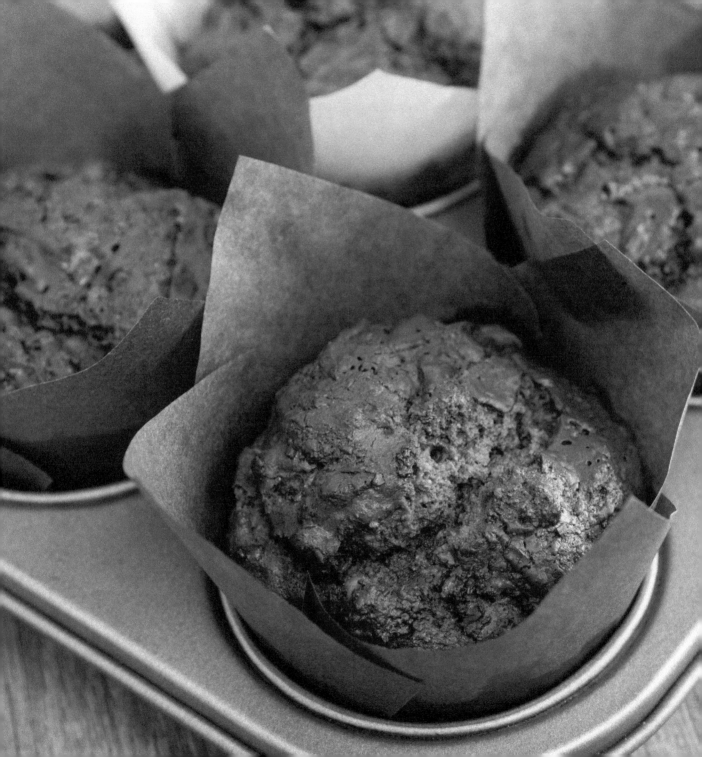

11. Chocolate, Quinoa & Zucchini Muffins

Serves: 8 | Prep Time: ~40 min |

Nutrition Information
(per serving)

- Calories: 354 kcal
- Carbs: 30.4 g.
- Fat: 19.4 g.
- Protein: 14.2 g.
- Fiber: 3.7 g.
- Sugar: 19.7 g.

INGREDIENTS:

- ½ cup dry quinoa
- 2 tbsp. coconut oil
- 1½ cups almond flour
- ½ cup walnuts (chopped)
- 2 large bananas
- ½ cup applesauce
- ¼ cup maple syrup
- ½ cup zucchini (shredded)
- 1 cup vegan protein powder (vanilla or chocolate flavor)
- ½ cup vegan dark chocolate chips (alternatively use cacao powder)
- 3-5 tbsp. almond milk
- 2 tsp. baking powder
- ½ tsp. cinnamon
- ½ tsp. vanilla extract
- ½ tsp. nutmeg
- pinch of salt
- ½ cup water (optional)

Total number of ingredients: 17

METHOD:

1. Prepare the quinoa according to the "Quinoa" on page 13 and set aside.
2. Preheat the oven to 400°F / 200°C .
3. Line an 8-cup muffin pan with baking cups, spray with coconut oil, and set aside.
4. In a large bowl, mix together the flour, cooked quinoa, nutmeg, walnuts, cinnamon, salt, and baking powder.
5. Take a second bowl and mash the bananas with a fork, and then combine the mashed bananas with the applesauce.
6. Stir in the vanilla, maple syrup, protein powder, and almond milk until all the ingredients are distributed evenly; if necessary, add the optional water.
7. Combine the separate mixtures into one large bowl. Stir until the batter is smooth and lumps have dissolved.
8. Finally, carefully fold in the shredded zucchini and chocolate chips.
9. Fill each of the muffin cups halfway.
10. Bake in the oven until the muffins are fluffy all the way through, for about 20 minutes.
11. Remove from the oven and cool for at least 15 minutes before serving or storing and enjoy!

STORAGE INFORMATION:

Storage	Temperature	Expiration date	Preparation
Airtight container M/L	Fridge at 38 – 40°F or 3°C	5-6 days after preparation	Reheat in pot or microwave
Airtight container M/L	Freezer at -1°F or -20°C	60 days after preparation	Thaw at room temperature; Reheat in pot or microwave

Note: Add extra chocolate chips or oatmeal flakes on top of the batter before baking for even tastier muffins, that are nutritious too!

Tip: If your batter seems too runny, consider adding less almond flour or water. If your dough is too dry, add more almond milk or water.

HHG Readers' Circle

Congratulations on your responsible and health-conscious decision to read this book.

We're grateful you've joined us and excited for your journey ahead.

We offer our readers the exclusive opportunity to become part of our readers' circle. Dozens of people are already enjoying *bonus* plant-based recipes and extra support on their journey to better cooking, meal-prepping, and weight loss (or gain, when intended).

Become part of our readers' circle today and get *The Vegan Cookbook* free of charge!

Simply subscribe to our newsletter and join hundreds of people with similar ethics and goals.

http://happyhealthygreen.life/about-us/evahammond/vegan-newsletter

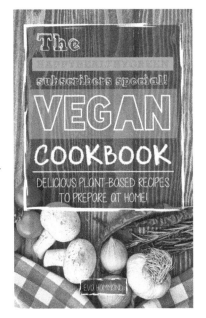

By becoming part of our readers' circle, you will receive our latest recipes, useful articles, and many more tips to stay healthy, right in your inbox.

Our readers enjoy unique support in their health plans and can always reach out to us for personal questions.

http://happyhealthygreen.life/about-us/evahammond/vegan-newsletter

Subscribe and become part of our readers' circle and get instant access to our unique *The Vegan Cookbook*'!

Enter your email address and let us help you stay committed.

Choose the plant-based lifestyle and renounce animal cruelty. **See you inside the readers' circle!**

**We hate spam and will never email you more than twice a week.

Conclusion

Can't get enough of these plant-based, high-protein recipes?

Learn how to prep protein-rich meals for the entire week from the comfort of your kitchen counter. Get started today. **Improve your physique, build muscle, and become the strongest version of yourself!**

Grab part two of the Vegan Meal Prep series that includes **91 recipes** and a customizable **30-day meal plan** (1600, 1800, 2000, 2500, & 3000 kcal/day).

https://www.amazon.com/Jules-Neumann

Note: some recipes in 51 Plant-Based High-Protein Recipes: For Athletic Performance and Muscle Growth are also found in Vegan Meal Prep: 30-Day Plant-Based High-Protein & Fitness Meal Plan.

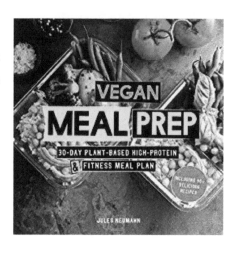

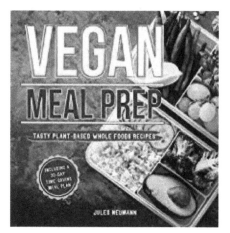

Alternatively, Part One of the Vegan Meal Prep series comes with **89 recipes** and a **30-day meal plan** that is applicable to different daily calorie needs (1600, 1800, 2000, 2500, & 3000 kcal/day). Rather than a muscle-building diet, this book and its recipes focus on trimming excess weight.

https://www.amazon.com/Jules-Neumann

If you have any questions regarding the Vegan Meal Prep series or any other book by Jules Neumann, feel free to send us a message at:

https://www.facebook.com/happyhealthygreen.life

Thank you

Finally, if you enjoyed this book, then we would like to ask you for a small favor. Would you be kind enough to leave an honest review for this book? It would be very helpful to both future readers and us!

You can send us your feedback by email or at our facebook page:

https://www.facebook.com/happyhealthygreen.life!

Did you discover any grammar mistakes, confusing explanations, or wrongful information? Don't hesitate to send us an email at:

info@happyhealthygreen.life

We promise to get back at you as soon as we can. If this book requires a revision, we'll send you the updated eBook for free when the revised book is available.

CPSIA information can be obtained
at www.ICGtesting.com
Printed in the USA
LVHW072238010120
642297LV00022B/2387/P

9 789492 788276